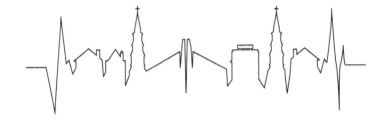

VITAL SIGNS
IN CHARLESTON

VOICES THROUGH THE CENTURIES FROM THE
MEDICAL UNIVERSITY
OF SOUTH CAROLINA

EDITED BY Carolyn B. Matalene & Katherine E. Chaddock

FOREWORD BY Raymond S. Greenberg,
PRESIDENT, MEDICAL UNIVERSITY OF SOUTH CAROLINA

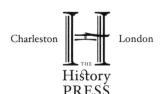

Charleston   London

THE
History
PRESS

Published by The History Press
Charleston, SC 29403
www.historypress.net

First published 2009

Manufactured in the United States

ISBN 978.1.59629.579.7

Library of Congress Cataloging-in-Publication Data

Vital signs in Charleston : voices through the centuries from the Medical University of
South Carolina / edited by Carolyn B. Matalene and Katherine E. Chaddock.
p. cm.
Includes bibliographical references and index.
ISBN 978-1-59629-579-7 (alk. paper)
1. Medical University of South Carolina--History. I. Matalene, Carolyn B. II.
Chaddock, Katherine E.
R746.S6V58 2009
610.71'1757915--dc22
2009026250

CONTENTS

FOREWORD

One of the most familiar sights in Charleston is a horse-drawn carriage loaded down with tourists. Traveling at the speed of one horsepower, these open-air vehicles afford a wonderful view of the beautiful houses and gardens that adorn our historic streets. Visitors can be seen gazing to the fore, aft, port and starboard as the charms of Charleston pass slowly by. The horses pulling these carriages have a more restricted field of vision, however, thanks to the blinders that adorn their harnesses.

Without intending any offense to these carriage horses, it occurs to me that university presidents share the same visual perspective. The focus of an academic leader is always trained straight ahead, thanks in large part to our own set of occupational blinders. Even at institutions with long and glorious histories, the president has to be more concerned about the road ahead than the route that was traveled in the past. I am no exception—my days tend to be filled with the future-oriented tasks of planning for new programs and facilities and securing the funds to make it all possible.

There is, of course, a great danger in never looking backward. Lord Byron wrote, "The best prophet of the future is the past." We at the Medical University of South Carolina, therefore, have every reason to celebrate the publication of this book by Drs. Matalene and Chaddock. They have given us a very insightful view of this institution, from its early days as one of the first medical education centers in the United States, through its struggles during the period following "the recent unpleasantness" to the thriving, complex organization that it is today.

What makes this account so authentic and honest is that it is expressed through the words of those who were participants in this history. These first-person accounts make us feel that we are listening to our predecessors describe the place and its people as they experienced it. While other histories of this university have been written and are laudable for their scholarly research, none quite captured the day-to-day life of our campus with the same richness of detail that Matalene and Chaddock infuse into their work. What we learn from this book, perhaps to our surprise, is that the experience of being a student of the health sciences has changed far less than the sciences themselves.

The nearly two centuries of the Medical University's history were a period of unprecedented expansion in medical knowledge. It is useful to remember that this institution was founded four decades before Pasteur advanced germ theory, seventy years before Roentgen demonstrated the imaging potential of X-rays and more than a century before Fleming discovered the antimicrobial effect of penicillin. One can only wonder at the number of times that curricula have been rewritten to keep up with the latest advances in scientific understanding. Through all of these changes, the constants have been the feelings of excitement, challenge, fear and frustration that greeted the first students on campus, as well as those who matriculate here today. Matalene and Chaddock have captured these emotions with rare clarity and poignancy.

For me, there is some comfort in knowing that the more things change, the more they stay the same. In the fast-paced world of modern healthcare, each successive generation of students is inclined to assume that those who preceded them could not have known the stresses and strains of mastering an ever-expanding knowledge base. In truth, while the "facts" that we teach have changed many times and become far more numerous and specialized, students have always faced a daunting challenge in absorbing the information of their day.

Arguably, the process of educating a healthcare professional is as much about being schooled in the culture of caring as it is about mastering any specific knowledge base. Although one may not be able to teach compassion or sensitivity, as our students observe their professors, hopefully they learn how to listen carefully, show respect for others and communicate clearly and honestly. Since the doors of this school were first opened, that has been a central part of our mission.

In that spirit, the words of Ralph Waldo Emerson seem particularly apt: "What lies behind us and what lies before us are tiny matters compared to what lies within us." Matalene and Chaddock have painted for us a portrait of what lies within many of those who have graced the Medical University over the years. Those of us privileged to be here today can draw great strength from the values that we have inherited from those who preceded us. We can only hope that these values will survive and flourish within those who follow in our footsteps.

Dr. Raymond S. Greenberg
President, Medical University of South Carolina
Charleston, South Carolina
June 2009

Acknowledgments

While working to recount the history of the Medical University of South Carolina through the voices of its key participants, we received invaluable support and assistance from dozens of current and past members of the university administration, faculty and student body. Earliest among those who would encourage and aid our efforts were MUSC President Raymond S. Greenberg and Alumni Affairs Executive Director Elizabeth (Betsy) Waters. We thank them with recognition that this volume could not have happened without their enthusiastic and essential support.

Additionally, individuals in numerous MUSC colleges and offices provided background information and pointed us to further resources for inclusion in this history. At the College of Nursing, our work was guided first by Dean Gail Stuart and then by Dr. Teresa Kelechi, Mary Lee Lavelle and Elizabeth Khan. Ann Brown, Lauren Smith, Catherine McCullough and Dr. Becki A. Trickey assisted our work at the College of Health Professions, as did Stephanie Oberempt in the College of Dental Medicine; Dr. Jeffrey Wong in the College of Medicine; Willette Burnham, Alicia Lockard and Laurine Charles in the Office of Student Programs; Bryan Moten in the Center for Academic Excellence; Sarah King, Kim Draughn, Susan Master and Ann Thompson in the Office of Public Relations; Dr. Steven W. Kubalak, *Humanitas* advisor; and Judy Holz in the President's Office. We are especially grateful to Tom Waldrep, Center for Academic Excellence, who continuously fielded our questions and offered expert direction throughout more than a year of research.

Those individuals who provided oral data through interviews, as well as written information from journals, letters, notes and even a blog, also contributed greatly to this volume. We extend appreciation for their contributions to interviewees Stephen Colbert, Dr. Edward (Eddie) Collins, Dr. Bernard Deas, Rosslee Green Douglas, President Emeritus Dr. James Burrows Edwards, Charlene Stuart, Dr.

Peter C. Gazes, Dr. Rose Delores Gibbs, Dr. William H. Golod, James Hodges, Catherine McCullough, Dr. Layton McCurdy, Dr. H. Biemann Othersen, Jr., Dr. Elizabeth Pilcher, Dr. K. Jackson Thomas, Dr. Edward (Ted) Welsh and Dr. Ralph Wilkie. Dean Mark S. Sothmann, College of Health Professions; Laura Cousineau, library program development and resource integration; Dr. Melissa J. Matthews Fussell and Dr. Anthony Colacino, College of Medicine; Andre C. Eaddy, the Graduate School, contributed written resources; and College of Nursing student Nick Porter shared portions of his blog.

To capture the events of the first century—more than half the history of MUSC—we relied on the tireless expertise of archivists who organize and protect documents of the past and who help researchers discover and recover texts. At the superb Waring Historical Library of MUSC, we were fortunate to have the assistance of Susan Huffius, Kay Carter and Dr. Curtis Worthington. Likewise, we benefitted from the work of E. Brooke Fox and Jennifer M. Welsh, who ably administer the University Archives. A group of archivists whose support has proved invaluable to our earlier research endeavors again provided their services: Henry Fulmer at the South Caroliniana Library; Harlan Greene at the Avery Research Center; Nicholas Butler at the Charleston County Library; and John White at the College of Charleston Archives and Special Collections. Additionally, we thank Jane McCrady Yates at the Citadel Archives and Museum.

Finally, we were fortunate to have the early encouragement and ongoing patience of The History Press commissioning editor Laura All, the precision of senior editor Hilary McCullough and the support of a dedicated and skilled research assistant, Amber Falluca.

A Note on Archival Editing

The letters, journal entries and other written records appearing in this volume generally are excerpted versions of the originals in order to allow space for numerous documents. Salutations and closings of letters are retained only when their wording connotes something of interest about the sender, recipient or context.

As editors, we retained as much of the authors' original writing styles as possible in the excerpts. We silently corrected only those spelling errors and small grammatical mistakes that appeared to be careless occurrences and might cause confusion for readers. When writers referred to themselves or others by first or last names only, we added full names when identification was not obvious and was possible. Additionally, we added class years of students when they were available and would assist in identification.

Carolyn B. Matalene
Distinguished Professor Emerita
University of South Carolina

Katherine E. Chaddock
Professor
University of South Carolina

CHAPTER 1

CHARLESTON NEEDS A MEDICAL COLLEGE

C harleston, South Carolina, has always inspired divergent views. From its founding in 1670, some visitors described an "unhealthy bog," while others insisted that it was bright, breezy and healthy. All agreed, however, on a variety of illnesses to contend with: epidemics of yellow fever and smallpox, cholera, malaria, dysentery, whooping cough and influenza. Natural hazards were common as well: hurricanes, earthquakes and fires, not to mention the large population of rattlesnakes as well as hostile Indians, some of them man-eating. And the sewage was forever contaminating the water supply. Perhaps, some argued, it was not the best place for a city since it was low and miasmal and the miasmal theory of disease was widely believed at the time. On the other hand, the tides did carry bad stuff away.

From the time that "Charles Towne" was founded, doctors were in great demand. But in the seventeenth and eighteenth centuries, what was a doctor? Some were self-styled physicians by virtue of a particular medical skill; some were surgeons who had apprenticed; some might be apothecaries or dispensers of drugs; some were no doubt quacks; and probably very few were trained and qualified physicians. Thus, one of the earliest issues in the practice of medicine was the necessity of establishing a procedure for licensing physicians, separating them from apothecaries and standardizing training. To that end, the Medical Society of South Carolina, the fourth oldest in the United States, was founded in 1789.

Members of the Medical Society, largely from Charleston though they intended to represent the entire state, met monthly in the following years to discuss such issues as meteorology, drowning, quarantine, leeches, clean water, yellow fever, fees and, eventually, the possibility of students. The minutes of the society report this motion by Dr. David Ramsay:

July 1, 1803:
Resolved, That this Society elect by ballot one of their Members to read Lectures on Anatomy, Surgery and Midwifery—and another to read Lectures on Chemistry, in the course of next Winter and that the Society will patronize the members so elected and use all their influence in procuring Pupils to attend their respective Lectures.

Although the lectures proved to be popular, this precursor would not become an official College of Medicine for another twenty years. The need for formally examining and licensing physicians was carefully explained by someone who signed himself "Aetius" and wrote a series of articles for the *Courier* in 1806:

The gentlemen of the law have very wisely guarded the Bar from the intrusion of ignorant or incompetent men, and oblige every person to study for a certain number of years before they are even eligible to be examined. On the contrary, every fellow wearing a black coat, a long face and a pair of spectacles, who has acquired impudence enough to pass for what he is not, and who can impose upon the ignorant by a specious display of a few technical or dog-latin phrases, or who by the smoothness of his tongue or the suavity of his manners can render himself agreeable, may assume the title of Doctor without being asked any questions about his education, and is at liberty to pick people's pockets even with their own consent.

In 1817, the Medical Society of South Carolina became a licensing board for the eastern half of the state; but still, there was no official medical college. The Medical Society was finally inspired to action when Dr. Thomas Cooper, the fiery president of South Carolina College in Columbia, gave an impassioned address to the Columbia Medical Board in December 1821. Cooper began with the familiar argument about the importance of keeping southern boys in the South:

A young man, bred in the southern climate of this state, and intended for a Physician, generally finishes his collegiate education at the age of about nineteen or twenty: he is then usually sent to New York or Philadelphia, to attend the Medical Lectures of the Professors there, for two or three years.
Let us review the circumstances of his temporary banishment...
He is sent a thousand miles from home.
He is sent to winter, in a northern climate: his health is exposed, and his constitution requiring to be acclimatized again when he returns south: forming a double hazard of health.

He is sent from the controuling eye of his parents and friends, exactly when he stands most in need of their anxious superintendance; when the passions are strong, the judgement weak, the propensity to pleasure almost unconquerable.

Dr. Cooper's comprehensive plan for a medical college suggested a Columbia location:

Situated as the State of South Carolina is, with a College already in prosperous operation—interfered with by no rival institution—what should prevent a medical school from being established at Columbia, upon a plan somewhat more eligible than the schools to the northward?

Let a Medical School be established, with a Professor of Anatomy; a Professor of the Institutes and Practice of Medicine; a Professor of Surgery and Midwifery; a Professor of Chemistry and Materia Medica, and Professor of Botany and Materia Medica—Five Professors.

Let the State allow to each Professor $1500 a year, for five years, by which time, I calculate, the school will be well able, at the usual fees, to remunerate its own Professors.

The Medical School may be put in operation entirely at Columbia, or it may be divided between Charleston and Columbia.

But Charleston doctors, the founders of the state's first Medical Society, were not about to let control leave town or be divided between Columbia and Charleston:

Minutes SC Medical Society
November 22, 1822
...It is our undivided opinion that such a measure, although the interests of the upper and lower counties might possibly be presented by it, destroy abroad the effect arising from contemplating it as one institution having all the energies locally concentrated.

The compelling reason was Charleston's abundant supply of dead bodies:

We think Charleston the most eligible first, because anatomy which constitutes the basis of the science cannot be effectively taught unless the means of obtaining Bodies are ample and easy. Anatomical preparation, public demonstration, as well as the [illegible] unequivocally point to Charleston as the place most likely to afford the facilities required.

The Medical Society carried its concern to the state assembly by way of a "Memorial" written by Dr. James Moultrie Jr., a leader in medical education through the century. The legislature approved Moultrie's Memorial without, however, offering financial assistance.

THE COLLEGE BEGINS—IN CHARLESTON

In 1823, the Medical Society of South Carolina became the official parent of the Medical College of South Carolina. Faculty members established and operated the school at their own expense, covering costs by selling tickets to their lectures. The college opened on November 8, 1824, with thirty students. The great event was memorialized in the *Charleston Mercury and Morning Advertiser*, November 17:

> This institution was opened on Monday the 8th instant at the new building erected for the purpose, at the west end of Queen Street in Charleston; the ground having been given by the City Council, and the other expenses having been borne by the professors. These professors were nominated and elected by the Medical Society of South Carolina, by whom the different branches were specified and assigned, forming the whole routine usual in Medical Schools.
>
> The week was taken up by the professors delivering introductory lectures within respective branches:
>
> On Monday, by Samuel Henry Dickson, M.D. Professor of the Institutes and Practice of Physic.
>
> On Tuesday, by Henry R. Frost, M.D. Professor of Materia Medica.
>
> On Wednesday, by Thomas G. Prioleau, M.D. Professor of Obstetrics and the Diseases of Women and Infants.
>
> On Thursday, by James Ramsay, M.D. Professor of Surgery.
>
> On Friday, by John Edward Holbrook, Professor of Anatomy.
>
> On Saturday, by Edmund Ravenel, M.D. Professor of Chemistry and Pharmacy.
>
> These introductory lectures were public and were attended not only by students who have been matriculated in this institution, but by a large number of literary and scientific gentlemen who crowded the lecture rooms with mixed feelings of pride and solicitude at the opening of this domestic institution under auspices of the talent of Carolina indulging the hopeful

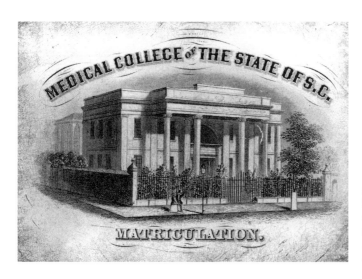

Queen Street
building before
the earthquake
of 1886. *Waring
Historical Library,
MUSC.*

prospect that our state will no longer remain in an entire state of pupilage to the learning and institutions of other countries.

In April 1825, the first class of five students graduated. Faculty minutes of May 2, 1825, draw attention to the reason for the fledgling school's superior location:

No place in the United States offers as great opportunities for the acquisition of Anatomical knowledge, subjects being obtained from among coloured population in sufficient number for every purpose, and proper dissection carried on without offending any individual in the community. Those impediments which exist in so many other places, to the prosecution of this study, are not here thrown in the path of the Student, public feeling being rather favourable than hostile to the advancement of the Science of Anatomy. In addition, the Southern Student can nowhere else receive correct instruction on the disease of his own climate, or the peculiar morbid afflictions of the coloured population.

Students typically began classes in November and finished in March. If they returned for a second year, they heard the same lectures of the previous year. The length of the academic year was determined it seems by the lack of refrigeration. Only in the winter months could the dissection of cadavers be tolerated. During their seven-month vacation, students were expected to work with their preceptors.

A medical student named Columbus Morrison, from Mecklenburg, North Carolina, kept detailed notes on the lectures during the academic year 1827–28 by Professor Samuel Henry Dickson:

The most diligent analysis of the air during the prevalence of an epidemic has never yet discovered to us any morbific matter. Some of the predisposing causes are also directly exciting causes as the morbific miasmas arising from decaying animal and vegetable remains, contagions, poisons. The others are merely exciting causes as intemperance love grief and all the passions of the mind. Since miasmatic effluvia is not always of that character which produces disease the term is objectionable and in place of the term malaria is adopted which at once expresses the nature of the effluvia...

The modus operandi of malaria in the production of disease is a subject now much in dispute. It is a prevalent theory that the malaria is taken in the mouth when we breathe and the saliva becoming impregnated with it is swallowed. Disease then begins in the stomach by sympathy or otherwise the whole system becomes affected. This theory may in some degree be true but that the action is chiefly through the medium of the skin we infer 1st from persons being more liable to its action during sleep when but little saliva is swallowed and the skin is most active.

(Dickson also covered the diseases and fevers of the day: intermittent fever, remittent fever, worm fever, remittent fever of children, yellow fever, catarrhal fever, typhus fever, spotted fever, pneumonia billiosa, hectic fever, angina pectoris, inflammations, hemorrhages, apoplexy, colic, gastritis, diarrhea, dysentery, cholera infantum, wormsbercular consumption, hepatitis, sore throat, pleuritis, bilious pleurisy, asthma, pertussis and rheumatism.)

THE GREAT SCHISM

The Medical Society had succeeded in standardizing training. But then the faculty of the fledgling school decided that the society was exerting too much control—especially in selecting faculty members. The quarrel began when James Ramsay was forced to resign his chair in surgery because of "public drunkenness." The faculty wanted Eli Geddings, the first graduate of the Medical College, chosen as his replacement, but the Medical Society elected John Wagner.

Thus began the great schism. Impassioned position statements were traded. Among them was this one from Dr. Edmund Ravenel, speaking for the faculty and addressing the Medical Society:

It is therefore apparent that the whole burden of establishing the Medical College has been borne by the Faculty—the various difficulties incidental to such an undertaking and under such circumstances, have been successfully overcome by the Faculty alone.

The College, with all its appurtenances and appendages, its character, its reputation, are the creation of the Faculty and the work of their hands. Is it not morally then entirely and exclusively the property of the Faculty? The Medical Society have contributed nothing but the name, they have even risked nothing, a failure would have ruined the individuals embarked in the enterprise, without a hazard to the society...The faculty claim the moral right of who shall or who shall not enjoy with them the privileges, honors and reputation, which have cost them the best years of their lives.

They therefore solemnly protest against any other views of this subject as oppressive and unreasonable.

After bitter recriminations, court battles and even new charters, for a time Charleston had two medical schools: the Medical College of South Carolina, overseen by the Medical Society, and the new Medical College of the State of South Carolina, chartered in 1832 by the rebellious and victorious faculty. Charleston, of course, could not support two medical colleges, so in 1837 the faculty of the Medical College of South Carolina all resigned and by 1839 it was reconciled with the breakaway school.

In November 1839, Dr. James Moultrie gave the gracious and conciliatory opening address:

I do indeed rejoice, not less as a member of the Medical Profession than of the Faculty, at the termination of our olden feuds, and at the hope, now that our ancient strife has ceased, that those who once have differed will again be united in the bonds of peace and amity, and in promotion of their common interests, usefulness and dignity.

A Doctor by Default

While their professors were quarreling, the students were dissecting. But J. Marion Sims, later to become a distinguished alumnus of the Medical College of the State of South Carolina, didn't know what to do next:

I graduated from Columbia College [South Carolina College] in December, 1832. I never was remarkable for anything while I was in college, except good behavior. Nobody ever expected anything of me, and I never expected anything of myself...

At that day and time, the only avenues open to a young man of university education were those of the learned professions. A graduate of a college had either to become a lawyer, go into the church, or to be a doctor. I would not be a lawyer; I could not be a minister; and there was nothing left for me to do but to be a doctor—to study medicine or to disgrace my family...

I said: "Father, I know that I have been a great disappointment to you...I suppose I must study a profession, so long as I have had a university education, and there is nothing else left for me but the study of medicine, if I *must* take a profession."

He said to me: "My son, I confess that I am disappointed in you, and if I had known this I certainly should not have sent you to college."

I replied: "I did not want to go; I knew that you were not able to send me there, and I knew that you would be disappointed, and that I should make you unhappy. I am sure that you are no more unhappy about it than I am now. But if I must study a profession, there is nothing left for me to do but to study medicine."

He replied: "Well, I suppose that I can not control you; but it is a profession for which I have the utmost contempt. There is no science in it. There is no honor to be achieved in it; no reputation to be made, and to think that my son should be going around from house to house through this country, with a box of pills in one hand and a squirt in the other, to ameliorate human suffering, is a thought I never supposed I should have to contemplate."

In the nineteenth century, future doctors typically worked for three years with a local physician before attending lectures at a medical school. Sims's father relented and suggested that he begin such an apprenticeship.

However, he told me to go and see Dr. Churchill Jones, and make arrangements to study medicine. The next morning I felt happily relieved at having been enabled to pass through that terrible ordeal with my poor disappointed father. I began immediately to read medicine with Dr. Jones. Dr. Churchill Jones was a man of very great ability. The people in the country around had very great respect for and confidence in him as a physician. But unfortunately, he drank. That for a time, seemed to unfit him for the duties of his profession. Besides, he had no facilities for medical instruction, for he had few or no books; and I read anatomy, read the practice, and all the medical books I could get hold of, without any teacher, or reading to any profit whatever. I was very glad when I was able to leave his office, and go to attend medical lectures. But he was a very great surgeon, and from him I imbibed a desire to distinguish myself in surgery, if I ever should become a doctor.

Sims entered the Medical College of the State of South Carolina in 1833 and stayed for one year:

I arrived there on the 12th of November, 1833...The Charleston Medical School [the Medical College of the State of South Carolina] was opened a very few days after my arrival, Dr. Samuel Henry Dickson was the Professor of Theory and Practice of Medicine. I well remember the introductory lecture; it was a brilliant effort, and I never heard such eloquence from a teacher's desk. He was a small man, very handsome, with a sweet, musical voice; a man of great literary acquirements, a fluent speaker, logical in his reasoning, convincing in his argument, and most captivating in his manner. But as a practical teacher I do not think that I ever learned much from him. The purity of his diction, and the eloquence of his discourse, and the beauty of his teaching captivated the ear, so that I was carried away entirely from the substance of what he attempted to instill into my mind. Wagner was Professor of Surgery. Holbrook was Professor of Anatomy, and he was a great teacher. He had but one equal, I think, as a teacher of anatomy, and that was Ballou, of Jefferson Medical College.

Sims soon discovered the essence of nineteenth-century medical studies: dissection:

I worked in the dead-house with interest. It was fascinating, and besides I derived a practical knowledge from it which I could appreciate, and could understand, and carry away, and know that I was doing something toward laying deeper the foundation for knowledge to come...

One night I was dissecting alone in the dissecting room, where there were ten or twelve dead bodies on many tables. I had found an anomalous distribution of the tracheal artery, and was anxious to trace it out. I had but a single candle. There was no other light in the room. I told Robert, the supervisor of the dissection-room, not to wait for me. I happened to knock

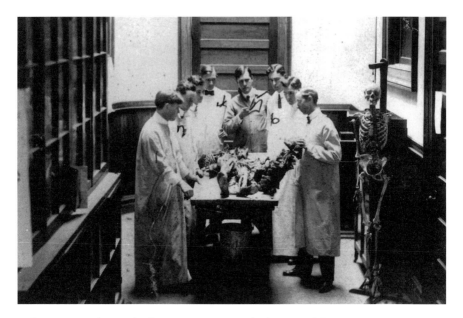

Early anatomy students and cadaver. *Waring Historical Library, MUSC.*

the candle over, and I was in the dark and had no matches. So I was obliged to desist from my work. I am not afraid of anything, but I must confess that I did not feel very comfortable as I threaded my way out in search of the door of exit.

And this reminds me of a similar experience of my friend Williams Sims Reynolds, of Charleston, when he was a medical student there in 1832. He was alone at ten o'clock at night, dissecting the parts concerned in an inguinal hernia.

A dissecting-table is about six feet long, and twenty inches wide, and thirty inches high.

To dissect the muscles of the abdomen, we place a billet of wood eighteen or twenty inches long and ten inches in diameter under the loins. This renders the muscles of the abdomen tense and prominent. This is increased by drawing the subject down toward the lower end of the table, so as to let the legs and thighs gravitate toward the floor, while the body is held firmly in place by a chain a yard long with a hook at each end. One hook is hitched in the scalp of the subject, and the other is hooked over the upper end of the table. If the hook should break loose the body would, by the weight of the legs, shoot over the lower end of the table. Reynolds's only candle was necessarily resting on the epigastric region of the subject. He had been at work all the evening on the right inguinal ring. He started to pass round the lower end of the table for some purpose, when he ran against the subject's projecting legs. This jostled the body so as to knock loose the chain at the upper end of the table, whereupon the body, having the roller billet of wood under the back, was, by the weight of the lower limbs, suddenly jerked to the floor in the upright posture, and its arms were forcibly thrown over Reynolds's shoulders. The light was of course put out. I think I should have left that body to the force of gravity. But Reynolds took it under the arms and replaced it on the table.

(Sims finished his training at Jefferson Medical College in Philadelphia. He returned to Lancaster, lost his first two patients and moved to Alabama. His specialty soon became women suffering from vesico-vaginal fistula. Experimenting in his own private hospital, he operated on slave women, over and over, until he transformed his bent spoon into what became known as the Sims speculum and devised the silver suture. One slave woman, Anarcha, underwent thirty operations before being cured. Although Sims's experimentation on slaves has been criticized by revisionist historians, he also has his defenders who place him in the context of the medical ethics of his day. He moved to New York City, starting the Women's Hospital, and spent the war years in Europe operating on aristocratic women, among them the Empress Eugenie, and being fêted by royalty. When he came back to Charleston, he was recognized as the father of gynecology.)

THE DUTIES OF A DOCTOR

Certainly, the physician's role was evolving throughout the South, and medical students were constantly being told of their responsibilities. Dr. Thomas Y. Simons, professor of the theory and practice of physic, in his introductory lecture at the Medical College in November 1835, offered this exhortation:

The life of a Physician is one of continued care, anxiety and study; no hour can he call his own. By night and by day are his services required, even the solemn day allotted by Almighty wisdom and mercy, as a day of rest to his creatures, is one of toil to him. But, how enlarged and elevated are his duties; what unbounded confidence is reposed in him, and with what gratitude and respect is he received and esteemed if he discharges, faithfully, his trust. He is

23

indeed the arbiter of life and death—and as his acquirements and capacities are circumscribed or extended, will he be a blessing or a scourge.

Dr. Samuel Henry Dickson, in his valedictory address to the class of 1841, also insisted on the moral superiority of physicians, even offering the first temperance lecture in Charleston to a perhaps unreceptive audience.

Your professional standing in society as well as your superior education will entitle you to give tone to the habits and manners of the circles to which you are to belong. Set every where the example of mildness, gentleness, and courtesy, mingled with a dignified self-respect. Fail not to denounce with all earnestness and on every proper occasion, the domestic and social use of the poison of the still, and thus strive to wipe away a deep and foul blot upon our national character.

Dickson also had strong opinions about concealed weapons:

Obey the laws, resist the wild and barbarous customs which in these evil times have been gaining ground so rapidly in the Southern and Western sections of this fair land. Leave to the Italian his stiletto—to the Spaniard his blood-stained knife, and to the Red Savage his tomahawk; but disdain even to seek protection against a ruffian by imitating him in the accursed practice of wearing concealed arms under whatever name and of whatever fabric. Die rather! And thus arouse the majesty of public opinion to aid a feeble legislation in avenging murder and according effectual security.

THE THESIS

From the college's beginning until the Civil War, every graduate of the Medical College of the State of South Carolina was required to write an inaugural thesis or dissertation to be approved by the student's preceptor and defended before the Medical Society or the faculty. The Waring Historical Library houses 1,858 theses, handwritten, some in elaborate script, on such popular topics as "On Intermittent Fever" (93), "On Bilious Remittent Fever" (60), "On Dysentery" (75), "On Malaria" (33), "On Tetanus," "On Gastritus," "On Typhoid Fever," "On Mania a Potu" (alcoholism) and "Delirium Tremens." A few interesting titles:

- Jones, Larkin G. 1829. "On The peculiarities of the Female, the physiological changes produced By Conception, and The treatment of some of the most important diseases consecutive to parturition."
- Eveleigh, Thomas. 1831. "On the Properties of the Xanthum Strumarium or Common Sheep Bur as an Antidote to The poison of Venemous Serpents."
- Hearst, John W. 1836. "The Properties, Uses and Injurious effects of Nicotiana Tabacum."
- Perry, Pope. 1837. "On the Professional Management of Negro Slaves."
- Mc Ree, Wm. Lucius. 1840. "On the use of Cold Water As a Therapeutic Agent."
- Agnew, Enid. 1845. "On The morbid effects of Intemperance upon the Animal Economy."
- King, Courtney S. 1853. "Yellow Fever as it appeared in Charleston during the summer of 1852."

CHAPTER 2

The Vibrant Years

The number of doctors in the South and in the whole country was rapidly increasing in the decades before the Civil War. And the Medical College was thriving. The catalogue for the Medical College of the State of South Carolina, the name it would be known by until 1952, listed the following faculty members for the session of 1845–46:

J.E. Holbrook, M.D. Professor Anatomy
E. Geddings, M.D. Professor of Surgery
S. Henry Dickson, M.D. Professor of Institutes and Practices
James Moultrie, M.D. Professor of Physiology
Henry R. Frost, M.D. Professor of Materia Medica
Thomas G. Prioleau, M.D. Professor of Obstetrics
C.U. Shephard, M.D. Professor of Chemistry

They were not, however, universally admired. Nor did the city of Charleston appeal to every medical student. Daniel A. Dobson, class of 1845, wrote to the Honorable Francis Bernard Higgins, senator from Newberry in the state assembly, evidently at the senator's request, and offered these critical commentaries about town and gown—with few commas:

Charleston, So.Ca. Jan 28th 1845
My dear Sir,
My time in town has not been on the whole progressing very agreeably. I don't see much to entertain—indeed attendance upon the lectures is sufficient to preclude almost all opportunities for amusement, few acquaintances are to be found and I do not make many among the students and none among the citizens and then everything I love in a country life is wanting here. I long to

eat some cornbread once more and to think of milk and fresh butter almost throws me into agonies but above all remember my miseries when you are drinking the fresh cool clear water. The trees too—oh for a sight of the pines on the way to Columbia once again! A slight glimpse of the dear beautiful red mud in Newberry streets would be refreshing too. In sober sadness tho' I have never in my life been so tired of a place as I am of this.

Some of my professors I am fond of but others I am half disposed to vote great bores.

Dr. Holbrook (Anatomy) is a rare man. His lectures are so full so clear so instructive and withal so unpretending and then never tedious that any man would be pleased to listen to him altho' he had never read anything of his science provided he have any desire to know how wisely how beautifully and how benevolently the good Creator has formed his creatures. Yet there is no affectation of religion in his Lectures neither does the Doctor make any pretension to piety or even very rigid morality.

Dr. Dickson, (Practice of Medicine) writes a pretty lecture and reads it well; but consumes a great portion of our time in discussions and speculations which we could very cheerfully dispense with—the more so as he will not get nearly thro his course in the manner he is pursuing. His notions of practice are drawn from extensive acquaintance with the best authors in the English French and German languages assisted by no trifling experience yet I fear too often warped and influenced by prejudices of so long standing that the Doctor (if aware of them) could not account for. He appears to be a very amiable and good man. Was married last week to a Miss Dupre.

Dr. Geddings is thoroughly acquainted with his art (Surgery) not only from industrious study of almost all authors of note and attendance upon the lectures and practice of the best surgeons of the world but also from a very considerable experience and to all this he adds a steadiness of nerve and a dexterity of hand truly to be envied by young surgeons. His lectures like Dr. Holbrook's are delivered without the aid of manuscript or notes and are to be commended for sound sense clear expression of his ideas a good style and happy selection of the most appropriate language. These three are the supports of the College.

Dr. Moultrie (Physiology) is a man not only learned but eminently so. He is even in some points in advance of the physiologists of the rest of the world. His lectures are full of thought evince deep study constant reflections and intimate knowledge of his particular science, but are written in the most strictly scientific style abounding in big words and dark abstrusities and delivered in the coldest driest most uninteresting lifeless manner. He is almost unanimously considered a great bore among the students.

Dr. Prioleau (Obstetrics) is excellent "in his vocation" writes a good lecture a bounding in good sense sound doctrine extensive knowledge of all writers on his branch conjoined with a great and well remembered experience. He is no doubt among the best of men—is a great favorite among those ladies who need his aid but among the students generally voted a bore, not so with me however.

Dr. Frost (Materia Medica) is well versed in his branch of Science and has also the benefit of much experience, but is admitted I believe on all hands to be a very poor lecturer. He seems more anxious than any other professor to gain the good-will of the students but is exceedingly unpopular among them in spite of all his efforts.

Dr. Shephard (Chemistry) I was much pleased with at first but my liking soon began to diminish and continued to do so until it was merged into dislike and this is constantly increasing. However he is not unpopular with the class. I believe him a good chemist but he is a bloodthirsty murderer of all elocution pleases himself in an astonishing degree in every thing he does and says. Has the most winning way as I conceive to gain dislike and in short is a genuine specimen of the produce of Connecticut.

Dr. Holbrook with scarcely an exception is a universal favorite with the class. He is something of an oddity too, tells a story inimitably, and has a straightforward hearty manner about him that every one is taken with. His Demonstrator in Anatomy Ogier however is as I humbly believe the greatest humbug in all the South. There is no professorship more important to the student than the station he is in if it were properly filled but I have heard nothing among the dissecting students this winter but one universal tone of dissatisfaction with Dr. Ogier.

...But upon the whole I believe they are superior to any other Faculty in the Union except perhaps the University of Penna. You may say this is a contradiction but my dear Sir it is not. There is no profession or calling as you are well aware which has more of humbug and quackery in it than ours and the fact of being raised to a chair in a College is not proof positive that a Doctor is an Aesculapious. I must beg pardon for my letter but since I began to write I've been to a fire—warehouse burnt on Magwood's Wharf—I have scribbled in a great hurry to get to bed.

Yours sincerely
D.A. Dobson

(Dobson graduated in 1845 and his thesis, "The skin as concerned in the causation of fever," was recognized as one of the three best that year.)

While Dobson was mostly impressed by the quality of faculty, a student named Frank Lumkins wrote to his friend and fellow student, Thomas McKie, in November 1851 and offered this less complimentary critique:

> Concerning this institution, I must say that my ideas of its merits—i.e., the capacity of its professors taking them in the aggregate—were vastly exaggerated and had I not taken my tickets so early I should have been tempted strongly to have gone on to Philadelphia and taken a perpetual ticket as you recommended. But before going I should have strove to extract a few teeth from our worthy janitor by a method as yet little talked of in surgery which necessity sometimes causes to be used upon the most unwilling patients. I used a few nautical phrases on him...
>
> Among the Professors there are none but two who are in any wise fit to lecture as far as delivery is concerned and these are [Professor of Chemistry C.U.] Shepard and [Professor of Medicine Samuel H.] Dickson. The others no doubt are very able men but they have a devilish poor way of showing it. [Professor of Pathology Eli] Geddings may do well when one becomes accustomed to his style but I think it more suited to a Methodist circuit rider than a professor in a medical college. Old [Professor of Physiology James] Moultrie turns his back on you and mumbles away and when he has consumed his hour he turns round to make his bow and seems to say "guess what I have been talking about." One out of the number who take his front seat may possibly say, but that is doubtful.

Dr. Thomas G. Prioleau, professor of obstetrics for forty-three years, also came in for criticism from a medical student writing to his mentor in Columbia:

Charleston, Nov. 16, 1853

Dear Doctor [probably S.L. Strait, who may have mentored this letter writer into Medical College]:

I reached the City near two weeks since, and would have complied with your request ere this, had I had the opportunity, but as you well know the effect it has on any person to change from a country to a city life, I am confident you will readily excuse my negligence. I have been attending the lectures some ten days, and I am pleased with all the faculty with the exception of one or two—which I consider very poor. Prioleau for example.

He takes up the whole hour in telling what a common man could make known in five minutes. I have not commenced dissecting yet, but I have witnessed the operations of the dissecting knife repeatedly. It is a "spectacle" to one who had never witnessed it, at first sight. I have not heard anything as yet that would interest you in this line of medicine. I saw your brother Richard in town today...

Benj. S. Lucas, Class of 1855

But everyone liked Holbrook. Dr. Holbrook had an unusual bedside manner, as recounted by that demonstrator in anatomy, whom Dobson thought "a great humbug," Dr. Thomas Lewis Ogier. Dr. Ogier read a memoir about Holbrook before the Medical Society of South Carolina in 1871:

Dr. Holbrook, as a practitioner, was very popular...The Doctor had some peculiarities or eccentricities, but these could be easily explained; for instance, his dislike to attend obstetric cases, or to perform any painful surgical operation. He never attended an accouchment in the whole course of his practice; and with his accurate knowledge of Anatomy, he never operated, if could get any one else to do it, in whom he had confidence...

His manner in a sick room was gentle and kind; but to those who did not know him well, sometimes seemed abrupt; for instance, where a patient was suffering from nausea, and seemed likely to vomit the medicine he had just administered, he frequently, without any notice, and regardless of bed-clothes, would throw a half-tumblerful of water in his face, and say "take that, and do not say anything more about throwing up." The patient would be momentarily startled, and protest against such treatment; but the nausea would pass off, the medicine be retained, and his temporary wrath against the Doctor would be changed to the feeling of gratitude and confidence.

One of his eccentricities was followed by a remarkable result. A young waiting man about the house was very liable to fainting fits. In brushing flies at the table he would often exclaim: "I am going to faint," and would, if not assisted, fall down in a swoon. The Doctor one day, whilst dissecting the digestive apparatus of a young alligator, called this boy to hold the parts for him, so as to keep the fibres. Just as the Doctor was most interested in tracing some minute muscular fibres, the boy cried out, "I am going to faint," and altered the position of his hand, and thus interrupted the dissection at a most important point. The doctor immediately gave him a sharp slap on the side of his head, saying, "well, go faint then, and come back quickly." The boy did as he was bid, and never fainted after this. He said he "was cured by holding the alligator."

(Perhaps Dr Holbrook's resistance to surgery was because of his true interest: herpetology. His five-volume study of North American herpetology was published in 1842 and widely praised, most especially by Louis Agassiz, the great naturalist of the age who held the chair of comparative anatomy in the 1852–53 session of the Medical College.)

THE CASE NARRATIVE AND MEDICAL PRACTICE

Case narratives were the way medical research was conducted and shared throughout much of the nineteenth century. This narrative, written by Dr. Robert Lebby, one of the Medical College's first graduates in 1826 and a public health official for many years, appeared in *The Charleston Medical Journal and Review* in 1848.

The story reveals his belief in the importance of local conditions as well as his willingness to use a vast array of potent drugs and harsh interventions:

"Tetanus occurring ten days after a Natural Labor"

The subject of this most interesting case was a highly accomplished lady, aged 25 years, of a nervous habit, light eyes, auburn hair and a very fair skin, indicating a strong scrofulous diathesis. She had three healthy children, and on the 12th May, 18___, at 9 o'clock P.M. I was called in...The labor progressed, and nothing occurred to interrupt the natural process, when, at 2 A.M. she was delivered of a son...on the 16th my patient was sitting up in her arm-chair. She continued to improve daily until the 20th, when she complained of headache, which was attributed to the confined state of her bowels; ½ oz castor oil directed to be taken...On 21st, two ounces solution of sulph. Magnesia...At 11 she was up and dressed—being a sultry day, the windows of the chamber were up—she remained sometime at her toilet, adjusting her hair, between two windows, when a fog came up from the sea, and this damp atmosphere passed directly through the room...

At 7 o'clock, P.M., she complained of headache and soreness of the jaws, with stiffness of the muscles of the neck...She complained of the right side of the neck and expressed great dread of lock-jaw. I endeavored to calm her fears, and prescribed 3i of paregoric, 3i of sweet spirits nitre, in a wine-glass of warm tea. Vol. Tinct. Of Laud. To be applied to neck and jaws, and foot-bath with mustard. 10 o'clock the stiffness of the neck increasing, inability to open the mouth, febrile excitement increased, pulse 100 and full. My patient was fully impressed that she had lock-jaw and would die. I bled her from both arms at the same time, until the pulse sank to 40 beats per minute, and administered a teaspoonful of laudanum, applied warm fomentations of hops to the angle of the jaws and neck, and repeated hot foot-bath with capsicum and mustard.

11 o'clock.—No improvement, repeated the laudanum and poltices of hop.

12 o'clock.—The mouth firmly closed, it was with great difficulty that a thin spatula could be introduced between the teeth.

Another doctor was called in who agreed with the treatment but suggested:

...as no advantage had been obtained from the lancet and opium, "to produce revulsion upon the system with the cold shower bath." The proposition was made to the husband and acceded to. Three or four buckets of cold water were thrown over the head, our patient being supported in a bathing tub. She was immediately wiped dry, enveloped in blankets, replaced in bed, and a 3i of laudanum, with great difficulty was administered. A profuse diaphoresis followed, mustard sinapisms were applied to the soles of the feet.

Even the professor was called in:

At 6 o'clock, Dr. Prioleau saw our patient with us, and suggested the use of tart. Emetic, 4 gr to 8 oz. water, a tablespoonful every half hour, until nausea and relaxation took place. I remained during the day and administered the medicine regularly every half hour, until 2 o'clock, P.M., when the two medical gentlemen arrived. Up to this moment, no effect whatever had taken place from the medicine, and no improvement in our patient. The medicine was continued, and a blister applied to the nape of the neck.

7 o'clock, P.M.—No improvement, and my medical friends agreed with me that our unfortunate patient was in a hopeless condition. The blister had not vesicated, and the antimony had produced little or no effect. It was determined the increase the quantity to 1 gr every half hour.

Unfortunately, the patient died:

> 10 o'clock P.M.—Nausea induced, the muscles of the jaws became perfectly relaxed, the mouth opened, and our patient attempted to vomit, when she screamed, sprang from the bed and immediately expired. Thus ended this melancholy but most interesting case...
>
> The conclusion arrived at was that the disease ensued from atmospheric influence, while our unfortunate patient was at her toilet, between the two windows, acting upon a moist skin, and a peculiar idiosyncrasy, favorable to a peculiar nervous irritability of habit.

(Although Dr. Lebby blamed the foggy weather and his patient's nervousness, it was later discovered that she actually died of tetanus contracted during a previous dental procedure.)

SEND MONEY: MED SCHOOL IS EXPENSIVE

Medical students, like all students, perennially worried about their finances. A.V. Carrigan wrote to his brother in Society Hill, explaining his predicament and his frugality:

> Charleston, Dec. 13, 1854
> Dear Bro., [to W.A. Carrigan, Society Hill]
> Your letter came to hand this evening which I was glad to receive. I can get on until Christmas with the clothing I have and then I'll only need a few shirts and some little things, you know a person's obligation to have. I have not spent a cent of money unnecessarily since I have been here. I have not gone to see anything which costs a cent. You expressed my opinion exactly in regard to going up Christmas. I had intended in this letter to have begged off, but you have saved me the trouble. We are going to get up a petition to have the lectures soon with the exception of one day or two. When I wrote I thought it would not cost more than $8 to go and return. I have got my diarrhea stopped. Will you write down to some of your trading houses to let me have a few articles along as I may need them. I need nothing that I know of but some shirts...I attended lecture tonight for the first since I have been sick. I went to the lectures every day but one...I hardly have time to eat, therefore you will excuse me for being brief...
> Your bro., A.V. Carrigan
> P.S. The remainder of my tickets will cost $70. The ticket office will be closed in 3 weeks.

Carrigan anticipated a lonely Christmas in Charleston without friends or holiday food, only firecrackers to mark the occasion:

Charleston, December 23rd, 1854:

Dear Bro.

...Things are as dull and monotonous here as walking around a tree. Our lectures close here tomorrow for a week and the boys are all feeling as good as they know how. The only part of me that rejoices is the sitting part of my body, which is greatly delighted at the idea of exemption from the hard benches for a week. We have plenty of subjects for Christmas. Chisolm's steam mill burst up night before last, and scalded and mangled together, some 4 or 5 persons, mostly negroes, all of whom we expect to get in a day or two. One poor fellow was brought in last night with all the skin scalded off him nearly.

I am now due two weeks board and part of another week—but that is not the object of this letter...It seems that the Post Master General has made arrangements to establish coaches from Charleston to Columbia, Augusta via several other points, which will exclude us here from communication with our friends. Now the thing I wish to suggest to you is this. Had you not better send me down money enough to buy my tickets before the arrangement ceases, with the South C. Road, lest I might not get it before the ticket office closes. And besides there is great uncertainty in those stage coaches anyhow. You know it would be less safe. I have borrowed $15 from my friend McCormick, and paid up to this evening. He will not need the money immediately...

The boys are beginning to get drunk at a sound rate. I hear nothing but fire crackers all the time. I reckon Christmas will see a heap of powder burned in Charleston.

My love to all. I have got no letters from any of our friends. Do write soon.

Yours affectionately, A.V. Carrigan

William Horn Battle, a graduate in 1858, wrote to his father in North Carolina on January 4, 1858:

Your letter with money came in very good time, for I have borrowed twenty dollars from McKay [probably A.M. McKay, class of 1858] & have not ten of that left. I have to pay a high price for board—have to buy my own firewood & light—have taken some private tickets and have had to buy, necessarily, more books, than I had any idea of. I shall be obliged to buy one more high priced one, & that, I reckon will be the last. I have tried to be economical—have not been to but one place of amusement since I have been in the City, where I had to pay a cent...But some how my money goes very fast...I will have to hand in with my "Thesis" thirty dollars ($30.00) by the 1st Feb. & will be much obliged to you sir, if you will send me more money by that time.

The professors of the Medical College of the State of South Carolina worried about financial support from the state. Dr. Eli Geddings, first graduate of the school and later professor of surgery, wrote to Governor John L. Manning to beg for more funding:

Sir,
...Thus far, although commencing under discouraging auspices with very slight patronage from the State and trifling assistance from the City, for which the Faculty rendered more than equivalent, the college has grown steadily in prosperity and reputation, until it has attained in point of respectability, an equal footing with the most reputable of similar institutions in our country. For this success, it has been mainly indebted to the untiring efforts of its Professors; for while other states have been most munificent in cherishing their Medical Institutions, South Carolina, although she has done something, has fallen far behind much of her sisters of the confederacy. In this age of active competition, this want of state patronage has placed us at great disadvantage, and at the present moment, especially when the rapid advancement of Science, growing out of the daily development of new truths, from new and complex processes of investigation, the appliances necessary in a thorough system of education and illustration, have become so numerous and expensive as to be entirely beyond the limited resources of a Faculty dependent exclusively upon the fees of students for their limited compensation...
Very respectfully,
Your Excellencies Obedient Servant
E. Geddings, M.D.
Prof. Of Surgery
Med. Col. State of So Carolina
Charleston 5th Oct. 1853

LOCAL HAZARDS

The first Roper Hospital on Queen Street was completed in 1852 as a city hospital and teaching hospital for the Medical College.

Gabriel Manigault had graduated from the College of Charleston in 1852 and, bored with life on the plantation, decided to go to medical school. There he learned about Charleston's scourge, yellow fever, up close.

> Charleston was visited by a severe epidemic of yellow fever during the summer of 1852, and in the month of October it was at its height...Neither Heyward nor myself felt any uneasiness about the fever, as we were natives and have passed through several yellow fever epidemics, and besides, I was a regular medical student since the preceding spring and I considered that it would be ridiculous for me to be running away from a disease which as a physician I would be obliged to treat. I therefore remained, and the next morning went to the Roper Hospital at 9, when the attending physicians made their daily visits, without allowing myself to feel that I was doing an imprudent thing...
>
> It was interesting to me to observe the fever patients at the hospital. Their color soon changed from yellow to mahogany, and the cracks in the skin all over the body through which the blood exuded were a feature in the disease for which I was quite unprepared.

There was also smallpox, sometimes leaving medical students homeless. Thomas J. McKie wrote to his "cousin" on December 25, 1853, from Charleston:

> Dear Cousin,
> ...I will now tell you of the predicament that I have been in (with three others) for the last three days. When I wrote you last I think I said that small pox was in the city; since that time it has reached the Planters Hotel, where I was boarding and has attacked so many that the proprietor was compelled to close the hotel, under the advice of professor [Eli] Geddings, and of course the boarders were shut out to get quarters elsewhere. We (four students) have been without a house for three days, eating about in spots and sleeping in porches. As we were from a house infested with the disease, we could not find but one house to take us in and at that house we are boarding and I hope temporarily. I never have been so much at a loss...
>
> I think it rather strange of Professor Geddings advising the proprietor to close the hotel and then tell all in the city who asked him not to take us in; which he certainly did. We think of going up the road until we meet the

down train, then get on it and go to some hotel and register from some other part of the country and in that way get board. It was certainly a rich time when we realized that only two of the four of us had money. I am happy to say I was one of the two. As we expect to have varioloia, we are determined to stay together so we can attend to each others wants.

...I can't say anything more of interest and therefore must close.

Yours Affectionately, T.J. McKie

I.H. Blair, a graduate in 1855, wrote to his friend, perhaps his preceptor, J.R. Mobley (class of 1844), about staying the course—in spite of smallpox and the incomprehensible Professor Moultrie:

Charleston, Dec. 26, 1853

Dear friend,

...There is a great deal of small pox here at present. I think it is almost over the whole City. A great many students have left on the account of it. The epithet that Prof. Gedding applies to those who ran away is d...d cowards. I don't think there will be more than one hundred and fifty students after Christmas out of over two hundred.

...I have seen several surgical operations since I came down. I saw Dr. Bellinger operate for stricture. Geddings has operated some few times; we have had Marshal Hall with us from London. He has been trying some experiments upon the Alligator before the class; I think he proved clearly the motor reflex action. He also gave us a lecture in Epilepsy which I have taken down in short hand; I will preserve it for you to see...I have not got home sick yet. I intend hanging on until the last lecture. I don't wish Geddings' epithet applied to me.

...I expect to dissect after today. I have dissected one arm since I came down. My turn has not come round yet, but I have got another arm from one of the students, I think best to dissect all that I can without missing lectures. The demonstrator is a splendid little fellow. We have recapitulations on anatomy, physiology, surgery, and obstetrics, also practice. Cain on Practice. Miles on anatomy and physiology, Chisolm on surgery, Lockwood on obstetrics. I visit the Alms House and Marine Hospital. The Roper Hospital is not open. There is some bad looking cases in the Hospitals. Professor Moultrie is one of the hardest cases that I ever met with for abstruseness. I haven't got the first single idea from him this winter. He must be a hundred years ahead or behind the times. I can't say which...

Yours, I.H. Blair

In spite of all the diseases, students did complete their two-year course of study and then fulfill the thesis requirement. Gabriel Manigault explained how he wrote his:

> When I returned to Charleston [in the fall of 1853] I resumed my medical studies and prepared my written thesis for graduation in the following March. The subject selected was "Venous absorption," about which I knew scarcely anything—and the consequence was that every thing that I wrote was copied out of some work on physiology. I was so unsophisticated at the time as to think that the production was a meritorious one, and I actually had the presumption to ask Dr. Moultrie, a few days before the distribution of the diplomas, to read it, as I fancied it to be worthy of the prize. The prize was awarded to a student named Gaillard, who was already of some medical experience. He was an able man, lost an arm while serving as surgeon during the war, and died lately (about 1884) at Louisville Ky.

THE COUNTRY DOCTOR

S.W. Leland, a graduate of the Medical College of the State of South Carolina in 1849, left his beloved hometown of Mount Pleasant to settle into the life—and the competition—of a country doctor at Mill Creek. His practice was not what he had expected:

> Another circumstance rendered my situation very unpleasant. The Physicians, who live on Mill Creek, depend very little upon the practice afforded by their neighbors, for the immediate vicinity is generally poor, and very healthy. The most lucrative practice is that afforded by the large plantations, situated on the border of the swamps and rivers, and for which there is great competition.

Dr. Leland quickly learned that succeeding in his practice meant treating slaves, just as Samuel Henry Dickson had explained to the class of 1841.

> Is the slave sick? It is his master's pressing interest that he should quickly be restored to health, and regain his fitness for labour. His place is not filled up, like that of the freeman, so called, by greedy competitors, so soon as he fails in the performance of his task. His sufferings are a loss, and his incapacity a positive burden to his owner, and every necessary and comfort are freely

provided that many conduce to his recovery. But it will be for you to point out and demand these means; it will be your office, full of gratification surely to minister to the wants of this inferior and thoughtless race of beings; and for their masters, I will affirm, that I have never yet been refused any reasonable requisition made in their behalf.

Dr. Leland waited for a call:

Day after day would I sit in that lonely house and wait in silent expectation for a "call," but no call would come. About once a week I would go to Columbia for a day, and refresh myself for another week of waiting. I would read until books became a weariness, and my medicines disgusting. My pride, in all the time never would suffer me to go and so solicit practice, and I say now in all honesty, that the practice which I did enjoy came to me, I never solicited it.

Writing in 1851, Leland recorded the events of his first years of practice—or lack of one:

1849
April 22nd Received my first call—The patient Frank a slave of the Estate of James Henry. Disease Hemmorhoids. I gained some reputation from this case, more from the manner of handling the tumours, than any thing else.

April 27th. Was aroused up at night to attend upon Fanny eldest daughter of Capt. L.G. Henry—disease Cholera Morbus. Made an impression in both of the above cases. Notified by both, that I would be their Dr. in future. These two cases completed my first months practice.

May 1st During this month I received two unimportant calls. Made nothing.

June 1st. A case of hocmatemesis occurring on the plantation owned by young John James Hopkins. A negro was sent to bring a Dr. Mayo, but being out of the way, I got the call, being the first I had received to a plantation. I treated the case satisfactorily to those concerned; and have ever since retained the practice. From being employed on this plantation, I gradually came into notice, and calls became less seldom.

July 23rd. Performed my first surgical operation. Protracting ball, from Adam slave of Gen. Wm Hopkins—shot by the overseer. I was not the regular physician on the place, but was sent for, because the attending physician could not practice surgery. I performed the operation to my entire satisfaction. None of the bystanders knew, that it was my first.

Soon, Dr. Leland made friends (if not money), found a wife and settled into his professional life.

1850

Jan. 1ˢᵗ. Have been practicing medicine nearly one year. I find upon casting up accounts, that my expenses have amounted to little more than $400. Cash received for services little less than $300, leaving a balance against me of $100. But I find myself tolerably well established, in my profession, and better prospects for another year.

Feb. 7ᵗʰ. Was invited by one of my neighbors (Arthur Reese) to attend his wedding over in Lexington. Having not much to do I determine, to go just for the novelty. Among the vast heterogeneous crowd that I met there, I was particularly struck with a young lady, by name Miss Sallie Edmunds. The liveliness of her disposition, accompanied with a peculiar elegance of manner, kept me by her side, nearly through the whole night. I enjoyed myself very much, and did not leave until after sunrise next morning.

Feb. Called upon Miss Sallie Edmunds, for the 1ˢᵗ time. I found that she was more attractive at home, than she was at the party.

April 25ᵗʰ. Invited Miss Edmunds to ride with me in the buggy. Before we came back, we were engaged to be married.

Oct 19ᵗʰ I witnessed this morning the death of Miss Elisa Cooper, eldest daughter of my host. She died of bilious fever, after an illness of 17 days. The grief of her parents can be imagined but not described.

Nov. 12ᵗʰ At the hour of 12 oclock I was joined in marriage to Miss S. Edmunds. My Father performed the ceremony. We were married in the old house.

CHAPTER 3

SUTURES AND SAWS FOR
THE CONFEDERACY

The Medical College suspended instruction from March 1861 to November 1865, the years bracketing the Civil War. Its faculty, graduates and students apparently determined that the South would go to war well armed with doctors in every extant field of medical practice and related research. Most of the faculty, including sixty-two-year-old Eli Geddings and sixty-nine-year-old John Edwards Holbrook, entered Confederate service, as did students and graduates. A few students, like Simon Baruch, decided to continue their education at institutions that had not yet halted classes—in Baruch's case, at the Medical College of Virginia, where he graduated in 1862.

Nearly four hundred Medical College students, faculty and graduates joined the Confederate cause. Many new doctors who were studying their anatomy class notes and practicing on cadavers only a year earlier quickly gained lifetimes of surgical experience. While they managed the constant need for suturing and amputating, expert medicinal botanists combed fields and forests for remedies to infectious ailments that invaded the camps. Physicians who walked pickets and loaded cannons one day worked in makeshift hospitals the next. Their enemies ranged from musket shot and cannonball wounds to pneumonia, measles, gangrene, yellow fever, typhoid and dysentery. Some fought disease and battle wounds in makeshift field hospitals; some joined in the battle itself; some divided their time between the forces guarding Charleston Harbor and service to the home community; and some older alumni contributed their instruments and supplies to the cause. A number of Medical College graduates spent many months in Union camps and jails as prisoners of war.

A STUDENT'S PRELUDE TO WAR

Watchful wondering about possible hostilities was a constant preoccupation among Medical College students after South Carolina declared secession in December 1860. With their careers and lives in the balance, students and faculty nervously weighed options of volunteering immediately for battles to come or waiting for possible resolutions short of civil war. One upstate student, James J. Palmer, from Echaw, wrote a daily diary during his first year of medical school in the months before the war. Excerpts provide an example of medical education intertwined with visions of military service.

January 12, 1861:
Visited the Roper Hospital after breakfast where I heard Dr. [Thomas G.] Prioleau lecture on auscultation and demonstrate on patients in the ward. Attended Dr. [Henry R.] Frost's lecture on Materia Medica. He is not very entertaining, being as nervous as a schoolboy in his first attempt at oratory, repeating sentences frequently. Did not wait to hear [Dr. James] Moultrie, Dr. Atkiss, as I thought I could do better at home reading, they being more prosy than Frost.

January 15, 1861:
She [his fiancée, Clemie] is very fearful that we are on the eve of a civil war and expresses her anxiety for the safety of those who are dear to her whose lives will be endangered in defense of their State—but, at the same time she does not wish me to hold back on her account and remain an idle spectator of an event in which we are all interested. I have determined upon consultation with my father not to volunteer until I know whether war will actually be declared. I have other duties which I owe to others as well as to myself to perform which I cannot neglect for the purpose in engaging in some useless military service or merely to enroll my name among volunteers for the considerable gratification of pride in other years. I can be of much more use to my country in years hence by close application to my studies than by wearing a uniform and doing camp duty for perhaps only a week or two. If our commissioners sent to Washington fail in their mission and Buchanan drives us to arms by refusing to evacuate Fort Sumter, I will then offer my service as a soldier.

January 17, 1861:

Attended Dr. Frost's lecture at 9 o'clock as [C.U.] Shepard was lecturing on a subject I had already seen demonstrated. I took that opportunity of walking to the P.O. where I was fortunate in finding a letter from Clemie [living near Spartanburg]...Like a true-hearted noble-minded Carolina lady she is willing to see me enter into the ranks in defense of our rights but thinks there is no necessity for exposing myself to danger at present or abandoning my studies. When war becomes inevitable she is then willing and anxious that I should take my part in the fray.

January 19, 1861:

Visited the Marine Hospital and went through the Wards with Dr. F. Porcher. There were three or four Spaniards in the Hospital who were as dark as mulattoes and at first thought they were but soon perceived a great difference between the two races. They all had very heavy eyebrows meeting at the nose and very bright black eyes. There was a young man from Edgefield who had been accidentally shot through the thigh—a member of one of the volunteer companies. He must feel very unpleasantly situated as he is of a respectable family and seems to be very intelligent and is now surrounded by all sorts of men—in the same room with sailors and Irishmen.

January 25, 1861:

I attended all lectures today...After dinner I went to the dissecting room where I remained until dark. I do not like Dr. [F.L.] Parker as a demonstrator. He seems to take it for granted that one knows more about the subject at hand than he should and consequently does not take much pains to demonstrate the minutiae.

February 6, 1861:

...Old Dr. Moultrie's benches were pretty thin this morning—many of the students having gone to the Races which are now going on. They did not miss much as I don't think anyone who heard him brought away any new idea unless it was that he was totally unfit for the position he occupies. Several times he faltered and seemed to forget the arguments by which to prove his points. I hope he will resign by the next year. Dr. Prioleau, Frost, and himself injure the College very much, I hear several students speak of going elsewhere next term.

Eventually, hostilities were inevitable:

February 9, 1861
   The news of the formation and adoption of the Provisional Government of the Southern States reached Charleston about 12 o'clock...This evening the news of the election of Jeff. Davis as President of the Southern Confederacy arrived, the President of the U.S. having flatly refused to come to any terms for the rendition of Fort Sumter. It is rumored that it will be attacked on Tuesday [February 12]. Preparations are long made with vigor.

Where There's a Battle, There's a Doctor

Being not just doctors and medical students, but Charlestonians first, a number of the physician defenders were ready and waiting at various fortifications around Charleston Harbor when the first shot signaled the start of the war. One of these, Francis L. Parker (class of 1858), was assistant demonstrator of anatomy at the college; by April 1861, he was stationed at Morris Island as an assistant surgeon while the town prepared for hostilities. Early excerpts from his hour-by-hour diary tell of a mix of strategy and confusion as Southern troops around Charleston Harbor battled to recover Fort Sumter from Federal forces:

12 April, 4 a.m. Action opened by a shell from Fort Johnson on James Island. The sound of mortar awoke all camps. The sentinels gave the alarm and fired their guns. Men were seen emerging in hot haste from their tents and running quickly to their respective batteries. Surgeons with bandages and lint in hand, with pocket case under their arms, with laudanum and chloroform and splints, all hurried to the posts assigned them. And now shell answers shell and batteries from the various points send back to each other their warlike sounds until the whole circle plays on Sumter, lighting up momentarily her guns' outlines... Sumter has opened. Crash goes her balls upon the iron battery and the 42-pound battery; they strike on houses and ricochet far out into the marsh and creek. Shot succeeds shot; now she answers Moultrie and is paying her regards to the floating battery. Our men are being made acquainted with the sound of balls—they are falling all about us. The action is general.
   10 a.m. Firing is perfectly regular, everybody is cool and calm...No one is hurt. Our men are getting used to the machine—a ball from Sumter comes, is buried in the sand or goes whizzing away into the marsh or up the Island; a moment after a hundred heads are seen upon our traverses watching for

another ball from Sumter. There it comes; "Look out" is the cry; down go our men, not a head can be seen, the ball has passed; up again we go, and so this continues...Our men watch with great interest every shot and mark its effect. Cries of that's a good one, hurrah for that one, bad, poor, try it again...

1 p.m. Sumter's casement guns dismounted or so injured that he has left the Morris Island side of the fort; he is combating furiously with Moultrie and the floating battery, and occasionally at Fort Johnson. The fleet has arrived, is now off the Bar. It numbers three steamships and one transport vessel—Pocahontas, Pawnee and Baltic—they are signaling Fort Sumter...

10 p.m. Tide going down, no signs of fleet, miserable cowards. [Major Robert] Anderson has just signaled them. They answer but remain inactive, calmly gazing at the battle; the execrations of our men are loud against them and yet our navy officers say their commander is brave—can it be so!—we doubt it...

13 April, 12:30 a.m. Just about us we hear the startling cry of sentinels, corporal of guard, bam! Bam! Boat traverses opposite Lamar's Battery; muskets are fired in quick succession...Leizeman's 24-pound howitzer belches forth, the grapeshot whistles over the heads of our men and splashes around the boat. It is now ascertained that there are but two occupants on board. These have thrown themselves flat in the bottom and vociferously cry, "Friends, Southern Confederacy, don't shoot for God's sake!"—again, the boat left to itself is carried down by the waves along the beach; now it is opposite Leizeman's battery...The musketting recommences, the frightened sailors cry lustily, "don't shoot, we are friends." The boat drifts unguided by the current, it approaches a second time the shore. Our men rush in and seize the two men, the causes of alarm. They prove to be two drunken fishermen who had brought two members of the Palmetto Guard to the Point in the afternoon—they had missed their way and attempted to land...

8:30 a.m. Our meal is over, we are lighting cigars when cheer after cheer reaches our ears. Out we run pell mell—Fort Sumter is on fire, hurrah, thousands stand on sand hills, embankments and traverses, the cheering is deafening...Now we have him—but no, there wave the Stars and Stripes towering above the flames and smoke, cries of what a gallant fellow Anderson is, his is all pluck, pluck to the backbone. And now the shot and shell fall like hail on Sumter. Every battery redoubles its fire...

10:30 a.m. Sumter still fires on Moultrie. Occasionally she pays her regards to the Floating Battery—flames are subsiding. Our efforts are directed towards the southern part of the building. The wind is favorable, if that part catches Sumter is ours.

1:30 p.m. White flag on battlements, hurrah! Cries of white flag, great cheering, she surrenders, wildest scene on Morris Beach, immense cheering, Hurrah for South Carolina!

(Dr. Parker served in the Confederate Medical Service for four years before returning to Charleston. He was later appointed professor of anatomy at the Medical College and served as dean of the faculty from 1891 to 1906.)

Dr. Robert Lebby Jr. (class of 1853) and Dr. William H. Prioleau (class of 1860) were among those whose training at the Medical College was put to use at the start of Civil War action, both serving at Fort Johnson on James Island during the surrender of Fort Sumter. Dr. Lebby was joined in wartime medical service by his father, Dr. Robert Lebby Sr., an alumnus of the second class to graduate from the Medical College, 1826. In a later memoir, Lebby Jr. helped resolve the controversy about who fired the first shot of the long war:

I was a resident and practicing physician of James' Island at the time the first gun was fired...and having been a college acquaintance of Captain [George S.] James, I was invited by him the previous day, April 11, to be on hand if anything transpired to require my services. I accepted his invitation and remained to witness the first, and last, gun fired at Fort Sumter at that time.

...As to the question of who pulled the lanyard of the mortar from which issued the first shell, there are only two living witnesses that I am cognizant of who were in the battery at the time of the fire, viz: Colonel Henry S. Farley and Dr. W.H. Prioleau. Colonel Henry S. Farley asserts in a letter to me that he pulled the lanyard by Captain James's order, and Dr. Prioleau asserts that Lieutenant Farley had charge of the right gun of the battery, and that the first fire was from that gun, Captain James giving the order to fire...Certain it is that either James or Farley fired it, but as Captain James gave the order to fire, it must have been Farley, as James would never have given himself the order to fire. I, therefore, conclude that Lieutenant Henry S. Farley fired the first gun at Sumter by Captain James's order.

SIMON BARUCH: FROM BATTLEFIELD TO FIELD HOSPITAL TO PRISON

At age twenty, in 1860, Simon Baruch traveled from Camden to Charleston to join 246 students at the Medical College, having arrived in the United States from

Germany only five years earlier. A year later, with the suspension of all academic activities, Baruch, who already had medical apprenticeship experience in Camden, managed to make his way to Richmond, Virginia. He graduated from the Medical College of Virginia in 1862 and immediately secured an appointment as an assistant surgeon in the Confederate States Army. He tended to the Confederate wounded, and a number of Union wounded, at the Second Battle of Manassas and Battles of Chancellorsville, Fredericksburg and Gettysburg. He was twice a Federal prisoner. Later, in an interview published in the *New York Times* (December 8, 1912), he explained his appointment:

> Every regiment was under the care of a surgeon, with the rank of Major, and an assistant surgeon with the rank of Captain. This latter was my office. The former established the field hospital in conjunction with other surgeons, while the latter was on the firing line with the regiment. There was a hospital steward in charge of medical supplies, these being carried in the medical wagon on marches, and a corps of litter bearers in each regiment. In the earlier part of the war the regimental band acted in this capacity; later, the whistling of bullets and shrieking of shells became substitutes for band music.

As a medical student only months earlier, Baruch found himself thrust into the position of practicing surgeon with great dispatch and some awe:

> On that day, Bull Run, my eyes beheld for the first time the tragical scene of a battlefield in all its overwhelming pathos. Mere remnants of men and animals; arms flung away in the mad retreat; blood pools that were less horrible than the shattered bodies with vermin at feast...Having left the medical school but a few weeks previously, and without practical clinical experience in surgery, it was my good fortune to have the privilege of visiting the field hospital, or rather temporary rendezvous, where during the battle of the two preceding days the wounded were operated on. Stopping in front of one of these improvised hospitals, I saw a burly surgeon standing ready to operate on a soldier who was being chloroformed on a "table" constructed of two barrels, upon which a door was laid. Surveying my slender figure and pale face with a glance of ironic contempt, the burly surgeon said, "Perhaps you would like to operate, doctor," stretching the knife to me with bravado. "Thank you," I replied and took off my coat, rolled up my sleeves, and proceeded with the amputation. It served to nerve me for the sad work that awaited me during the three years following.

At Boonesboro, Maryland, Baruch was ordered to care for the wounded at a makeshift hospital in a church yard while Confederate troops fell back in retreat. He later recalled making do and becoming a prisoner:

> When I made my first rounds of my "hospital," seventy-five seriously wounded men lay on the floor...An operating table was erected on the lawn—two barrels and a door, the door obtained from an adjacent house abandoned during the battle. The patient was chloroformed, and placed upon this rude table. I proceeded with my work...The rattle of musketry pierced the peaceful air, followed by the clattering of a thousand hoofs and the discomforting spattering of bullets upon the upper walls and roofs of the houses round about us. In a few moments the streets of Boonsborough were filled with galloping cavalrymen. I realized that I was a prisoner!...Two months were spent in Boonsboro as a prisoner. They would have been the most delightful of my war experiences by reason of the courtesies of the Union medical men and the social amenities to which some lovely Maryland "sympathizers" of the gentler sex materially contributed, but the delightful days were marred by an illness which deprived me of many of the latter.

Released in Baltimore, Baruch was captured again in the summer of 1863 and sent to Fort McHenry in Baltimore Harbor until a prisoner exchange was negotiated. His summary judgment:

> When the true history of the civil war is written, after all passion has subsided, it will be found that there were genuine chivalrous men on both sides, and that any lapse of manhood or fairness must be ascribed chiefly to unavoidable circumstances, and rarely to intentional cruelty.

His son, Bernard Baruch, later recalled:

> The war left an indelible influence which remained with Father for the rest of his life. Let the band strike up "Dixie," and, no matter where he was, he would jump up and give the rebel yell...I have seen Father, ordinarily a model of reserve and dignity, leap up in the Metropolitan Opera House and let loose that piercing yell.

HOMETOWN HEROICS

Many of the Medical College's alumni physicians barely left home during the war. Instead, they managed hospitals around the harbor where sick and wounded from North and South joined the usual group of citizens needing medical care. Dr. Edward H. Kellers (class of 1858) served at the Negro Hospital in Mount Pleasant, at Fort Sumter and at Fort Moultrie. Entries in his diary tell of life as a wartime Confederate surgeon balancing family, including a wife and infant son in Charleston, with medical duties:

> May 31st [1864]: Sat on medical board. Received order giving me temporary charge of Negro hospital at Mt. Pleasant.
>
> June 5th: Visited city. Saw Dr. Ogri [probably Dr. Thomas L. Ogier, Medical College class of 1830, and district surgeon in the Confederate army]. Heard from him that Dr. Moore of South Carolina Artillery was in charge of my hospital and I to remain as assistant. Have to be satisfied though I think it is not treating me with justice...
>
> June 11th: Reported for duty to Sullivan's Island...In attendance to hospital at Mt. Pleasant...The bodies of Cols [Lawrence M.] Keitt and [O.M.] Dantzler were brought from Virginia June 8th and buried near each other at Orangeburg County.
>
> June 16th: Enemy shelled by hospital. Had red flag flying. Hauled it down and replaced yellow one. Discontinued firing before the yellow was put up...General artillery practice in the harbor.
>
> June 17th: Visited Mr. Marchand's servant. Enemy fired at a steamboat returning from Sumter. The shell came within 50 yards of where I was standing with my wife.
>
> June 22nd: Amputated the right leg of Anthony, a servant of Mr. [illegible]. Took it off at the point of election. Purchased 10½ buckets of salt. Paid $300 for operation.
>
> July 1st: Visited city. Received a basket from Midway. Saw in the city Mary and Sally...
>
> July 2nd: Enemy attack James Island...Enemy on Battery Island. Blake lost two guns.
>
> July 3rd: Enemy attacked batteries at Fort Johnson and repulsed by our troops under Col. [Joseph A.] Yates. The first South Carolina A manned the batteries...
>
> July 19th: Enemy kept up a furious fire on Fort Sumter all day...

July 23rd: Visited city. Dined with Allen. Saw Yankee prisoners playing baseball corner of Rutledge and Broad St. Weather very pleasant...

August 3rd: Exchange of 50 Yankee prisoners for 50 of our officers.

Friday, 7th October: Since I have written continuing my diary, I have had some prisoners to attend at the hospital. They are treated as friends having volunteered to work on government work. The prevailing diseases now are Remd Fever and dysentery, yellow fever in the city quite fatal...My mother and brother paid me a visit.

Monday, 10th October: Visited city. Dined with Allen. Bought sole leather $35. Had first case of yellow fever in hospital from 32nd Georgia Volunteers. Died.

November 10th: My family started for the plantation. The weather was delightful. Had a quick passage to the city...My wife and I promenaded the city. News in the city that Sherman had evacuated Atlanta laying it in ashes. Purchased gloves, $50.

November 18th: Rose at five o'clock. Had everything ready for the cars which leave at six o'clock. Saw my wife and child safely on board. Weather still fine. Saw a case of variolous in Negro hospital. Expect to be sent to Fort Sumter...

December 1st: Today I received orders to accompany the 32nd Georgia Volunteers to Pocotaglio. Surgeon Porcher [probably Edward G. Porcher, class of 1860] is put in my place at post hospital. Last night I went wrecking to steamer Pocatese which ran aground on Drunken Dick's Shoal...Got several articles: beef, sugar, rope...Left for Pocotaglio the next day...Received orders to go to Coosawhatchie. Traveled all night. Next morning found they met the enemy between Polo and Cusa. Cadets, 47th Georgia Volunteers and King's Company of regulars. Fought all the morning, but the enemy succeeded in drawing our skirmishes. Our loss was 2 killed and 18 wounded. I set the field infirmary near the railroad and sent A.L. Taggett with the ambulance corps. Rain dreadfully all day. Was exposed to the weather. Next day was skirmishes...Our loss was 2 killed and 10 wounded...Reported to Surgeon Ogri on the 10th. He gave me furlough for 24 hours. Visited my family. Found all well. Arrived at Mt. Pleasant on December 15th, 1864. Reported to Dr. Moore although which is to be done with me is in the dark.

December 15th:...My horse has been nearly starved during my absence. Got some fodder for it...Received orders to report to Fort Moultrie on temporary duty until Dr. Geiger returns from Fort Sumter. Like the change very well and have nothing to do here...Rumor says that Savannah has been surrendered to the enemy today.

December 19th: The flag of truce ended today at ten o'clock. The enemy have not shelled either the city or Sumter. Today is the anniversary of my wedding day. Had the house in Market St. repaired where a shell had passed through. Weather warm and fine.

Saturday, 31st:...This ends the year. Our confederacy is still existing and resolved upon securing her independence. She has met with many reverses lately, but these will only tend to nerve her army to more glorious deeds. God grant that the close of the coming year may meet us enjoying the blessings of peace.

Thursday, February 16th: Orders were issued today to prepare for evacuation. Charleston and the islands are to be given up and we are to concentrate on the interim of the state...My old home is to be left in the hands of strangers, and they my enemies. What a sad thing it is.

(After the war, Kellers remained in Charleston to become a druggist and a general physician.)

BEETS, SHOOTS AND LEAVES

Medical College graduates in the field throughout the Confederacy were indebted to their fellow alum Francis Peyre Porcher (class of 1847 and later a professor at the Medical School) for compiling and publishing a lengthy reference volume aimed at instructing Confederate doctors to use the bounties of southern plants and trees as medicinal sources. After graduation, Dr. Porcher practiced and studied in Europe before returning to Charleston to help found the college's preparatory school, to operate a hospital for African Americans and to edit the *Charleston Medical Journal and Review.* Published in 1863, his *Resources of the Southern Fields and Forests* became an essential and comprehensive guide for Confederate physicians who found themselves low on supplies. Porcher, however, had even more expansive uses in mind for his comprehensive guide, explaining in the preface:

> I trust that after the war shall have ceased there will still be no diminution in the desire of every one to possess a source from whence his curiosity may be satisfied on matters pertaining to our useful plants. The Regimental Surgeon in the field, the Physician in his private practice, or the Planter on his estate may themselves collect and apply these substances within their reach, which

are frequently quite as valuable as others obtained from abroad, and either impossible to be procured or scarce and costly.

Among the hundreds of nature's remedies and palliatives suggested in the volume were:

Bené (Sesamum)—The planters and farmers throughout the Confederate States should save and cure all the leaves of the Bené now growing, to be used in camp dysentery, in colds, coughs, etc., among our soldiers, in place of Gum Arabic or Flax Seed. One or two leaves in a tumbler of water imparts their mucilaginous properties.

Dogwood (Cornus Florida)—Since the war, the bark has been employed with great advantage in place of quinine in fevers—by physicians in Sumter District, S.C., and elsewhere—particularly in cases of low forms of fever, and in dysentery, on the river courses, of a typoid character. It is given as a substitute for Peruvian barks.

Thoroughwort, Bone-set (Eupatorium perfoliatum)—Thoroughwort, drank hot during the cold stage of fever, and cold as a tonic and antiperiodic, is thought by many physicians to be even superior to the Dogwood, Willow, or Poplar, as a substitute for quinine. It is quite sufficient in the management of many of the malarial fevers that will prevail among our troops during the summer.

Quercus falcata. Spanish oak...This is possessed of the astringent qualities characterizing the genus; it has not, however, the purgative property found in the Q. tinctoria. It is employed as an astringent wash for gangrene. A decoction is administered with great success in dysentery, pulmonary, and uterine hemorrhage, and some have said, in intermittent fever.

Nepeta cataria, L. Catnip. Natural in upper districts; collected also in St. John's; vicinity of Charleston...Employed in popular practice in colds, asthma, amenorrhoea, chlorosis, hysteria, and the flatulent colic of infants; in the latter condition this herb is universally employed. It was also used in yellow fever...An infusion of the flowers was said to open obstructions of the liver and spleen.

Sassafras. Two or three leaves, dissolved in water, yield a mucilaginous drink. I made great use of the tea prepared with sassafras root, gathered extemporaneously, while Surgeon to the Holcombe Legion, S.C. Vols. It was given whenever a warm, aromatic, mucilaginous tea was required, in fever, pneumonia, bronchitis, catarrhs, mumps, etc...A cheap and wholesome beer for the use of soldiers, or as a table beer, is prepared from the sassafras, the ingredients being easily obtained. Take eight bottles of water, one quart of molasses, one pint of yeast, one tablespoonful of ginger, and one and a half tablespoon of cream of tartar, these ingredients being well stirred and mixed in an open vessel; after standing for 24 hours the beer may be bottled and used immediately.

Beta vulgaris. Beet. Vinegar is quite important to us in the present exigency. The following method will enable us to supply the place of imported vinegar: the juice of one bushel of beet, which is easily obtained, will make from five to six gallons of vinegar...Wash and grate the beets, and express the juice in a cheese-press, or in any other way which a little ingenuity can suggest; put the liquor into a barrel, cover the bung with gauze, and set it in the sun, and in fifteen or twenty days it will be fit for use.

A Surgeon's Field Manual

Precocious J. Julian Chisolm was only twenty years old when he graduated from the Medical College in 1850 and twenty-eight when he became professor of surgery at his alma mater. He observed battlefield surgery during a year in Italy and was present to care for the wounded at the Battle of Fort Sumter. The surgeon general of the Confederacy, Medical College alumnus Samuel Preston Moore (class of 1834), requested his service in authoring a volume that became the indispensible instructional guide for surgeons operating in tents and open air. His 1861 reference work, *Manual of Military Surgery, for the Use of Surgeons in the Confederate Army: With Explanatory Plates of All Useful Operations*, attracted enough demand to merit two more editions during the war. In chapters ranging from "Flap Amputation of the Leg" to "Rupture of Abdominal Viscera," Chisolm used experiential examples to help battlefield surgeons. Typical of his vivid descriptions from his own observations and experiments was this discourse in his chapter on "Treatment of Punctured Intestines":

In examining the archives of surgery we find cases in which portions of the intestines have been cut off, the cylinder of the bowels reunited by sutures, and excellent recoveries obtained. I have recently had under my care a lunatic, who, some months since, attempted suicide by opening his abdomen, drawing out his bowels, and completely severing two feet of intestine. Dr. Gaston, of Columbia, S.C., who had the case under charge, brought the two open ends of the intestine together, and securing them by carefully-arranged sutures, returned them within the cavity. The patient made a perfect recovery. This accident, which terminated so successfully for the lunatic, suggests an operation for a crushed intestine, which may offer better prospects than leaving the bowel to sough and form an artificial anus.

Pain management, a constant concern at field hospitals, elicited this advice:

Opium...will ever be the greatest boon to the military surgeon. It allays both local and general irritation, annuls pain, soothes the mind, blunts the sensibility of the injured nerves, and quiets the tumultuous action of the heart...It is therefore a remedy that should never be absent from our reach. Of all the preparations of opium, morphine is, perhaps, the best article for wounded men...The rapidity of action when morphine is used endermically is a very great advantage on the field, where every moment is of value. For complete narcotism, where a sufficient quantity of morphine is used, five minutes are all that is required; while with chloroform we all know that, when under excitement, its inhalation is often extended to from twenty to thirty minutes, and even longer—time which the surgeon in the field can not well spare.

Wound dressing and care, an ongoing difficulty for patients, nurses and doctors, was the topic of this warning:

The surgeon should never be in haste to change the cold for warm application...A more effectual mode of keeping down reaction is by using ice bladders, which are placed upon the india-rubber, waxed, or oiled silk covering...Whenever ice is used, never apply it directly to the skin, but always through the intervention of compresses. When possible, these bladders should be of india-rubber or gutta-percha...The animal bladder is a miserable substitute, as it is not only a very dirty application, allowing the water to ooze out and keep the patient constantly wet, but the bladders soften and decompose, becoming very offensive, and are soon destroyed.

(One of the few surgical innovations credited to the Civil War was "Chisolm's Inhaler," a compact nasal inhaler with two nozzles to accurately direct chloroform. In 1868, Chisolm left Charleston for Baltimore, Maryland, where he became dean of the University of Maryland Medical School, founder of the Presbyterian Eye and Ear and Throat Hospital of Baltimore and a contributor of scores of articles to medical journals.)

CHAPTER 4

SLOW RECOVERY...WITH PHARMACISTS, NURSES AND FEMALE DOCTORS

The years of Civil War aftermath marked times of unmatched struggle for the Medical College. When it reopened in 1865, pent-up demand kept the size of the student body barely respectable for a few years. But soon full-time professors were assessed $100 each to keep the school running; and by 1871 only six doctors comprised the graduating class. In 1872, graduates numbered a record low of two. Both lack of available financing and increased competition from a flurry of new medical schools, including diploma mills with no students, hindered the struggle to stay alive.

The Medical College was down, but not out, as it slowly increased graduating classes throughout the final two decades of the century. Its rebirth was aided by the arrival of two distinctly new groups of students in those years: pharmacy students and female students. Nursing students arrived in 1883, and although their training school was initially only loosely affiliated with the Medical College, their presence was felt in classes taught by Medical College faculty and in hospital duty beside Medical College students.

ODYSSEYS AT WAR'S END

Gabriel Manigault (class of 1854), who had been held prisoner at Fort Delaware, started for home in early 1865. On the way he found two of his medical school professors:

> Doctors Miles and Chisolm were fellow travelers the day that I went from Chester to Charlotte and their pleasant company enlivened and shortened the journey. Dr. Miles had seen his brother at Chester and reported him as saying that the prospects of Lee's forming a junction with Johnston were very slim...

The early ending of the war was to us three no longer a matter of possible doubt. It was sad to think that so many sacrifices had been made in vain, and we could clearly see that the whole tone of southern society would be changed in consequence of our failure.

Dr. Chisolm considered that southern defeat would not affect his prospects to any extent. He was certain of his ability to earn a living by his practice wherever he was, and he had no strong attachments to any place. He would try Charleston as a field of labor as soon as he could return, and if he saw no prospects of succeeding there he would go elsewhere without worrying much over the necessity for the move.

Dr. Miles was strongly attached to his native State and the city of Charleston where he had lived since boyhood and where he had risen to fame. He had desired to be simply a professor at the Medical College of the city, where, as a gifted lecturer, he would have attracted many students, and he could easily have made an income of $4000. With 200 students in attendance, each paying $20 for the annual course. He had been so bent on this as his future that he had neglected altogether the practice of his profession...

I was of course strongly attached too to the old order of things in South Carolina, and although I had studied medicine had allowed ten years to pass without attempting to practice it. I was therefore unfit even for the attempt, and at the time I could see no future for myself except to return to the Cooper river rice plantation and see whether the new order of things would permit me to maintain myself there. I had this advantage over Dr. Miles, that I had a home in Charleston to which I could go, and where I could consider at leisure what I would do.

(All three travelers settled into academic life after the war: F.T. Miles to a professorship in anatomy at the Medical College of the State of South Carolina, Gabriel Manigault to the faculty of the College of Charleston and J. Julian Chisolm to the Medical College and then the dean's chair at the University of Maryland Medical School.)

Doctor John Lawrence Ancrum (class of 1860), who had been first a Confederate navy surgeon but switched to the army after his ship was captured, ended his wartime service by walking home from Tennessee. Years later, during his final illness, he wrote to his friend Dr. Henry B. Horlbeck (class of 1859) and recalled those times:

1900
Abbeville S.C. Saty.17
Dear Harry:

As you see I am still on my back and getting no better fast...[During the Civil War] I was chosen out of over 150 surgeons in or in reach of Atlanta, and given charge of all the hospitals from Atlanta down to SW Georgia, and I was absolutely too young and too innocent to realize the great distinction and compliment thus paid me...Then I went to Morgan's command when I had a hell of time until with Bill Davis (Tim's brother), Basil Duke and others we laid down our swords on the Tennessee mountains and wandered back on foot to my wife and child, mother and sister, amid the ruins and ashes of Columbia, with $30 in gold pd. me by Mr. Cochrane for attendance on Hy Young thro a desperate case of double pneumonia there, I wagoned my way to Charleston with all my dependants, where living in two rooms I made my own fires, helped cook, and trudged around on foot for a year to get a bone at market, or the scant loaf of bread that served our frugal meal, this was 1866.

A DETERMINED RESUSCITATION

Against formidable odds, on October 12, 1865, the medical faculty, including Professors Eli Geddings, James Moultrie and J. Julian Chisolm, reorganized and reopened the school after its four-year closing. The books were mostly gone, the records and minutes mostly destroyed and the equipment damaged. And there was, of course, no money. Wax models from the museum were even sent to New York to be sold. But the school was in session, and on April 12, 1866, this hopeful notice appeared in the *Charleston Courier*:

This time-honored institution is evidently undergoing a process of vigorous rejuvenation...Important changes of organization, whose benefit it requires exclusively professional judgement to appreciate, have been enacted...We feel assured that the increased advantages, not surpassed by those of any other Medical Schools in the country, and equaled by but a few, must attract a larger class than ever before thronged its lecture rooms, or studied the specimens in its extensive and choice Museum. We are glad to learn that the latter was uninjured by the bombardment, and that but few of its specimens have been lost.

The students at the last session numbered thirty-four, which, considering the unusual disadvantages to which the College was subjected, was very encouraging. Out of this number thirteen were graduated.

On January 15, 1867, student Henry W. DeSaussure (class of 1867) took notes from Dr. Chisolm's lecture. Like many other doctors returning from battle, Dr. Chisolm was able to teach from extensive experience:

Contused and lacerated wounds. For a limb extensively torn up, muscles skin and arteries, nerves are torn across, the skin being tough is extensively torn up, the vessels contract while the tendons and nerves hang out like cords. Muscles are sometimes torn from one of their attachments. Amputation necessary to prevent the traumatic gangrene which must follow. Gunshot wounds are of this nature but are dry, 2ry hemorrhage following in 8 or 10 days more frequently. Such wounds attended with tremendous shock. Patient becomes cold with great mental depression and thirst easily overcome by encouragement and stimulants. Death from primary hemorrhage even from a large vessel very rare, 2ry much more common. When a patient is brought 1st indication is to examine wound while patient is in collapse and part paralyzed. Wound should be explored by probing, and the finger is the best probe. A firm probe can make the wound as long as probe giving false impressions. Catheter is next best if finger too large. Having found bottom of wound look for foreign bodies whether they be ball or any other mechanical irritant.

When classes began in November 1871, only three full-time students attended. The college had no money. But rather than close the school, the faculty passed two resolutions:

April 22, 1872

Resolved, That in consideration of the present condition of the many worthy young men anxious to adopt medicine as a profession, to meet the usual expenses incident to such study—we deem it advisable to recommend to the Board of Trustees the propriety of opening the college during the coming winter as a *free school*, open to all worthy applicants whose preliminary education may in the opinion of the Faculty have fitted them for so responsible an undertaking.

Resolved, That with a view of increasing the facilities for education and thus promoting the best interest of the Profession, we further deem it advisable that the college term be extended one month, and that the number of professorial chairs be increased by instituting that of Gynecology.

No tuition was charged until 1876 and attendance rose, though not to prewar levels. From 1876 to 1900, an average of twenty-one doctors graduated each year, with a low of twelve in 1892–93 and a high of forty-three in 1900.

One of the students during those lean years was Henry Tracy Ivy (class of 1880), a native of Louisiana, who had apprenticed to Dr. W.D. McDuffie in North Carolina before starting classes at MCSSC. He kept a careful diary of academic and social events during his first days in medical school:

Monday, Oct. 14, 1878

In Charleston, So Ca at 4:30 A.M. Stop at Hilton's house, sleep til 7, then down to breakfast. Then promenade over the city. Walk til 10 A.M. Negro Parade Day. At 2:40 P.M. call on Dr. J.P. Chazal, who chats with me awhile and recommends a boarding house. I commence boarding with Mrs. Hodges and a pleasant place it is too, tho pretty steep.

Tuesday, Oct. 15

At breakfast at 8 A.M. Write to Ma, Alice, and Florence. To college at 9 A.M. and listen to lectures til 1½ P.M. Dr Chazal & I go to Bank of Charleston and I get draft for 200 dollars—cashed. Deposit 100. Pay my matriculation fee and commence generally. At 4 P.M. walk up to St. Mary's Church and call on Father Northrop. Promenade in the city. Home to tea at 7.

Wednesday, Oct. 16

To college at 9 A.M. Gynacol-clinic at 10. Michel on Physiology at 12. 1 P.M. presented my letter of introduction from Dr. Wood of Wilmington to him. Bot Fowne's Chemistry and ordered Gray's Anatomy and Dalton's Physiology. Promenaded to Artesian Well. Went over the Museum. Home to tea at 7...

Friday, Oct. 18

To college and after to walk. In the dissecting room, see the first subject, a Negress. Late in evening call on some of the boys. Home to tea and read awhile. Buist gave us a clinic of a sailor who in a storm was caught by the top sail and kept there many hours. Upper part of thigh broken.

Saturday, Oct. 19

To college 9. In the hospital at 12. Kinloch operated on a man for stricture of the urethra complicated with vesico-scrotal fistula and scrotal abscess. We stayed in the hospital til nearly 3 P.M. Then I went up to Mrs. Parks. Dined at 3:30, then back to dissecting room. Scruggs and Wilheard & myself walk to the Battery & home...

Sunday, Oct. 20

Breakfast at 9 A.M. At 10 David, McDow and myself board the Sappho for Sullivan's Island. Walk on the beach to upper end of same. Eat oysters on half shell. Back to Fort Moultrie. We get into the caves thro a small window at the sally port. See Osceola's grave. In the boat at 6, to my house at 7, having walked over 14 miles and sailed the same. After tea I go to Mrs. Parks, home at 10 P.M., then to bed.

Monday, Oct. 21

Buy my dissecting instruments of Dowie and Moise. Sent off letter to Grandma. My last day in my present boarding house & I hate to move. But $5.00 per month is an item to me, you bet. Rained in afternoon and I didn't move as I expected to, can't say I want to. Not feeling particularly well today...

Wednesday, Oct. 23

Attended lecture. Raining. Abscess of the mammary gland. Gynacol-clinic in afternoon. Did my first dissecting. Arm and thorax of woman—stay in dissecting room til night. Home to tea. Chat awhile then up to my room...Dissecting is deuced dirty work. We have a fat subject...

Friday, Oct. 25

Feel o.k. this morning. Pay Mood $5.00 on the board after clinic. Otis Kinloch, five others and myself cut lectures and went yachting. Went to Morris Island...Had a glorious time. Lunch on board. Back at 4 P.M. to dissecting room and work til night...

Monday, Oct. 28

To college as usual. Letter from Preston; & photo. After arrive to dissecting room. Finished upon the brachial plexus and axillary space. After tea walked around on King Street with David. Bot me a pair of Florida Beau Cuff Buttons $1.00. Then to home. Study til 1½ then feeling sleepy crawled in.

Thursday, Oct. 31

To lectures as usual in morning. After dinner smoke awhile, then to Dissecting Room. Simons never found any fault with me this time, you bet. At 7 we went to chemistry quiz, after came by the Charleston Hotel & heard Wade Hampton speak.

Friday, Nov. 8

Up at 7, feel all o.k. Study a while in afternoon. At 4½ to hospital and served with a Jury of Inquest composed of medical students on the body of a Negro. The Coroner and Jury were medical students and Dr. and assistant were M.D.'s making the medical men in the party. Mood & I went body snatching—got in at 12:30. Raised a woman & a baby.

Thursday, Dec. 19

To College. On Jury of Inquest over Garvey—suicide—arsenic. At night to Shepard's quiz & lecture on the spectroscope. After went to hospital with Rhett and had a good time with him til 10. Letter from Florence.

At the end of the diary, Ivy left some memoranda:

Charleston Medical College, Oct. 21ˢᵗ. Am having a jolly good time and know more than when I came to this place. And besides enjoying myself, think I will learn as much as in any other place I could go to. Anyhow am going to try. The boys here are a jolly set and I am in with the liveliest of the lot.

Dr. Walter Peyre Porcher, son of the eminent botanist and doctor Francis Peyre Porcher, earned his medical degree in 1881 during those precarious times. But his father's fame didn't help Porcher remember what he read:

At the end of the two-year course [at Union College] I returned to my native city and entered the medial college for the regular three year curriculum. During my first year at the medical college, everything being new to me, it seemed impossible for me to retain anything. Everything seemed to go into one ear and out of the other. I attempted to read a medical book and I forgot the beginning before I got to the middle and I forgot the middle before I got to the end. It seemed utterly impossible for me to comprehend the whole field of medicine even with my father's assistance, who constantly aided me with his knowledge and advice. Thanks to a merciful Providence the same inspiration and guidance came to me at this juncture which has been with me all throughout my life.

Finally, it happened that there was a student in the class who was too poor to buy books, but I noticed that he wrote a very clear hand and took elaborate notes on the lectures. It occurred to me at once that herein lay the key to the solution of the problem. Take notes, study the lectures, and give back to the professors on examination, as near as possible their own words.

Professional Nurses: "A Great and Widespread Need"

Many concerned Charlestonians noted that training schools for nurses were springing up in other states but missing in South Carolina. Bernard O'Neill, chairman of the commissioners overseeing Charleston's City Hospital, pointed to the intersection of opportunity and need in a report published in the *Charleston City Yearbook* of 1882:

> The school [for training nurses] has to be located in Charleston, for only here are there a large number of sick persons brought together for treatment, and of course, where instruction can be given. Elsewhere, this employment is held in such respect that ladies of good family connections seek this education and after graduation find remunerative employment in the best homes in the country, and are treated with the highest consideration.

The Charleston City Council and the South Carolina General Assembly approved funding, and the first students entered the South Carolina Training School for Nurses in 1884, launching the endeavor that would eventually evolve into the School of Nursing of the Medical College of the State of South Carolina. They confronted a residential, two-year course of study with lectures; nursing duties; and rules, rules and more rules.

Nursing was demanding work if you could get it. The 1883 application form indicated that only the right ladies need apply:

1. Candidate's name in full, and address
2. Condition in life, single or a widow
3. Present occupation or employment
4. Place and date of birth

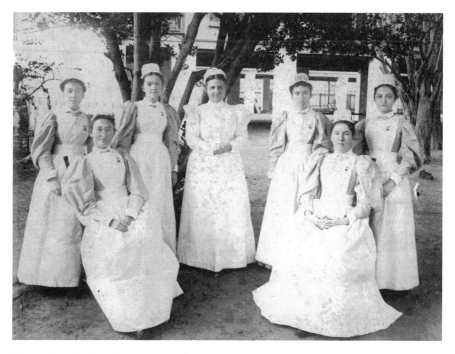

Nurses, class of 1897. *Waring Historical Library, MUSC.*

5. Height
6. Weight
7. Where educated?
8. Are you strong and healthy, and have you always been so?
9. Are your sight and hearing perfect?
10. Have you any tendency to pulmonary complaint?
11. Have you any physical defects?
12. If a widow, have you children? How many? How old? How are they provided for?

The teaching listed in the 1883 prospectus was to be in the hands of "visiting and resident physicians and surgeons," largely those associated with the Medical College. The major areas of required learning were described as:

1. The dressing of blisters, burns, sores and wounds; the application of fomentations, poultices, cups and leeches.
2. The administration of enemas, and use of catheter.
3. The management of midwifery, and uterine cases.

4. The best method of friction to the body and extremities.
5. The management of helpless patients; making beds; moving, changing, and giving baths in bed; preventing and dressing bed sores; and managing positions.
6. Bandaging, making bandages and rollers, lining of splints.
7. The preparing, cooking, and serving of delicacies for the sick.

Then there were those rules! Rules about activities in the "home," on the second floor of the City Hospital, found their way into the prospectus:

Rules for the Home:

Rule 1. The hour for rising is 6:30 A.M. Before leaving the Home for the Hospital, each nurse must make her bed, dust and arrange her room and closet, leaving them in good order, so that they may be ready for inspection by visitors at any time during the day. The hour for closing the Home is 10 P.M. All inmates of the Home are expected to be within doors at that hour, unless they have special permission to be absent...

Rule 2. The hours for meals are—breakfast from 7 to 8 A.M.; first dinner, 1:30; first supper, 7; second supper, from 8:10 to 8:45. Nurses must not linger in the dining room after meals...The parlor is for the reception of visitors, but a nurse can invite ladies to her room if agreeable to her room-mate.

Rule 3. Conditions upon which the nurses can have the privileges of the laundry: Twelve pieces, well marked, and one dress are allowed each person per week. No laces, muslins, or white muslin skirts will be received...A book with list of clothes, dated, must be sent in every week, with name on the outside of book...

Rule 4. The nurses are under the authority of the Principal, in the Home, in the Hospital, and when on private service. When taken off duty, on account of sickness, they must not leave the home nor return to their Hospital duties without the direction of the Principal...

Rule 5. A Physician will be selected by the President of the Board to attend the nurses in sickness. They will not be allowed to consult any other medical man without permission from the Principal...

Rule 6. Nurses who may have children will not be allowed to keep them at the Home.

Commissioner O'Neill had prevailed in initiating training for nurses in Charleston, but his vision of a pipeline of trained nurses for City Hospital had fallen short. In the *City Yearbook* of 1885 he complained:

The Training School...has not been kept as was first intended, to the strict betterment of hospital service, but rather as a school of instruction for pupils educated at the expense of the City, with the ultimate view, after acquiring a useful profession, to seek service in private medical practice in this and other cities, stimulated by the hope of lucrative employment...Although there are already eight ladies ready to receive their diplomas as trained nurses, the Commissioners of the City Hospital after making the entire outlay for their education from the City Treasury have no claim whatever upon them for their services in the interest of the sick poor of the city.

(The first nurse training school in Charleston closed in 1886, just a few months before the earthquake partially destroyed the hospital in which it had operated. A second training school would arrive in 1895.)

THE GREAT QUAKE OF 1886

The Medical College was gradually regaining its enrollment when disaster struck again. Dr. Francis LeJau Parker, appointed demonstrator of anatomy in 1859 and eventually dean from 1892 to 1906, described his up-close experience with the earthquake:

9:51pm August 31, 1886

I had just reached a point on Tradd street, opposite Mr. Lewis F. Robertson's garden gate, when I heard a roaring sound apparently in the direction of James Island Cut, which was southwest of where I stood. I made up my mind that a cyclone was coming, and instinctively turned towards the direction indicated, confidently expecting to see the air filled with the flying debris from James Island. Seeing that the sky was perfectly clear, I stood awaiting developments, when I heard another and louder roar coming from the northwest. I then began to feel the vibrations of the earth very distinctly, and realized that they were produced by an earthquake. From that instant the vibrations increased rapidly, and the ground began to undulate like a sea. The street was well lighted, having three gas lamps within a distance of two hundred feet, and I could see the earth waves as they passed, as distinctly as I have a thousand times seen the waves roll along Sullivan's Island beach. The first wave came from the southwest, and as I attempted to make my way towards my house,

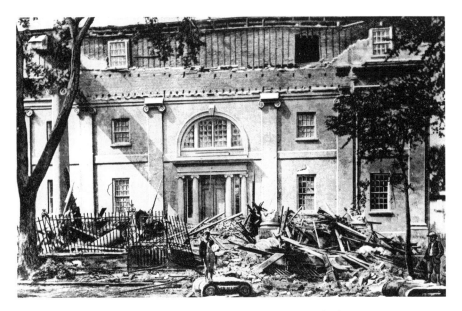

Earthquake damage to Queen Street building, 1886. *Waring Historical Library, MUSC.*

about one hundred yards off, I was borne irresistibly across from the south side to the north side of the street. The waves seemed then to come from both the southwest and northwest and crossed the street diagonally, intersecting each other, and lifting me up and letting me down as I were standing on a chop sea.

I could see perfectly and made careful observations, and I estimate that the waves were at least two feet in height. In order to make my way along the street, I had to tack, so to speak, from one side to the other...When I had reached a point in front of Dr. Fraser's residence, I saw the high brick wall between his house and the house of Mr. Parker Ravenel reeling from west to east, and am sure that it leaned over at times as much as 40 to 45 degrees from the perpendicular. At this moment one of the chimneys of the house on the opposite side of the street came crashing down in front of me. The greatest violence of the shock was over before I reached my house.

The earthquake damaged the Medical College buildings so severely that wooden buildings had to be hastily constructed and classes held in the Marine Hospital. The legislature appropriated funds for repairs and classes resumed on campus for the spring of 1888.

FITS, STARTS AND FINALLY PHARMACISTS

By 1867, the Medical College provided "students desirous of becoming graduate apothecaries" with two courses (chemistry and material medica), an exam and a designation of "Graduate in Pharmacy." However, it was not until 1881 that a formal Department of Pharmacy was approved by the state legislature. The annual announcement bulletin of 1882 proclaimed:

> For a long time it has been felt, especially by the Pharmacists, that instruction in matters relating to their branch was inadequate in the State, and the Pharmaceutical Association in conjunction with the Medical College urged upon the Legislature the necessity of making further provision in this direction. At the last Session of that body it enacted an amendment to the Charter of the Medical College empowering it to create a department of Pharmacy and to confer degrees in that science...This department has thus been established and for the present will consist of a Professor of Chemistry, a Professor of Materia Medica and Medical Botany, a Professor of Practical Pharmacy, and an assistant of Pharmaceutical and Practical Chemistry.

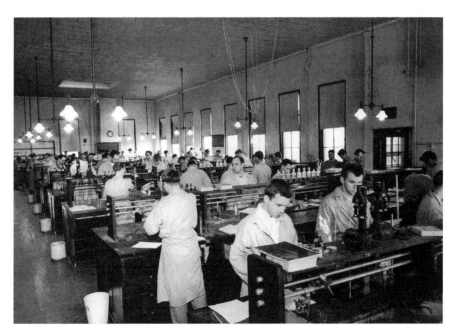

Students in pharmacy laboratory. *Waring Historical Library, MUSC.*

The first graduates of the new department did not face a high academic bar, according to the "requirements for graduation in pharmacy" stated in the 1882 bulletin:

1st. The applicant must be of good moral character.
2d. He must have worked two or three years in a pharmacy.
3d. He must be nineteen years of age.
4th. He must have completed two courses of instruction in this or a similar institution, the last of which must have been in this department.
5th. He must have passed a satisfactory examination.

The fledgling department closed in two years for lack of interest and funding. It bounced back in 1894 with renewed academic rigor and a commitment to allowing a new kind of student: female. The 1894 bulletin reported:

This department has thus been re-established, and for the present will consist of a Professor of Chemistry, Urinology and Hygiene, a Professor of Materia Medica and Therapeutics, and a Professor of Practical Pharmacy. Requirements for students: They must attend two courses in the pharmaceutical laboratory, and must have worked two years in a pharmacy before entering the College, showing a certificate of the same. They must pass a satisfactory written examination, and shall be twenty-one years of age. Instruction in the chemical and pharmaceutical laboratory is graded, and consists of a junior and senior course. These courses are designed to fit the student to conduct the processes of manufacturing and dispensing in the most thorough and economical manner. Women are admitted as students.

THAT OTHER EARTHQUAKE: WOMEN IN WHITE COATS

The timing was right, the women were ready and the Medical College faculty agreed:

Faculty Minutes, March 20, 1894:
    Dean read a communication asking if female student will be admitted. DeSaussure offered following Resolution. Buist 2nd. Adopted.
    Female Students. Resolved: That the dean be requested to answer the communication of J.C. Fulman saying that this college will accept female students.

At the meeting of May 31, 1894, the time had come for a vote. The matter was discussed, and Professor Buist offered the following resolution, which was adopted:

> Resolved: That in the opinion of the Faculty of the Med. College of the State of So. Ca. The time has come for the opening the doors of the Medical College to Female Medical Students to be instructed both in Medicine and Pharmacy and that to accomplish this purpose they announce the fact in the annual catalogue. In so much as there is some difference of opinion as to the consent of the Br'd of Trustees to this course the Dean be requested to see the members of the Br'd and ask their concurrence in this "action" ("unanimous action") of the faculty as conducing to the interest of the college by placing it upon an "equality with other institutions."

Evidently the board concurred—perhaps because of financial considerations. The treasurer reported that of the $1,275 owed by students, $300 had been collected; therefore, there was now enough money to run the college in the fall.

COEDUCATION IN THE CLASSROOM

Joseph Taliaferro Taylor attended the Medical College for the full three years, graduating in 1899 as valedictorian. He wrote to his sweetheart, Anna Cuthbert, in Summerville with great frequency, including the news of women as fellow students.

> March 18, 1897
> ...Well, I must say goodbye as I have to go to the college and hear some of the last fond words of our professors. I do wish so much that you could go with me. I learn that some girls are going to attend next year. Now is your chance.

And indeed, some girls did attend the next year. Taylor took note:

> Oct. 4, 1898
> Just as I was going to write early this morning, a student came around to ask me to go to Dr. Parker's office and assist him in an operation, which I did. We operated on a small boy for granulation of the eyelids and the boy had to take chloroform. Then I had just time to catch a car for the hospital.

Two girls sit just above and back of me at the clinics and every time I move, I bump the back of my head on their knees. They always ask me to excuse them, which I do. They seem as composed as can be.

In two or three years there will be a whole stack of them at this college. I thought that I would not like their presence, but I find that I do not notice their presence in the least. One is a Miss [Emilie] Viette and the other one Miss [Rosa] Hirschmann (a jewess).

Oct. 6, 1898

...Our work at the college goes on just as if we had never had a holiday and everything is quite natural, except the girls there. It seems strange sometimes to look around and see them there. I have not seen one of them blush since they put in an appearance. Had they done so at times, they would have been perfectly excusable. At least, I think that they would. They must have quite a supply of nerves, so they should at least make good surgeons.

Nov. 3, 1898

...Miss Viette and James are now great chums and she gives him flowers every morning.

Nov. 10, 1898

...Two Italians have a bear out in the street just in front of the house and they have him doing all sorts of things. He was at the college yesterday, but it is my opinion that he will not be brought there again soon, as the students played too many tricks on him by giving him indigestible food.

Dec. 5, 1898:

It has been getting steadily colder here all day and I know that it will be real crisp and nice in the morning, but I shall nearly melt from ten until two as that time will be spent at the hospital where it is always dreadfully warm and close. Just add to these conditions a surplus of chloroform, ether, iodoform, carbolic acid, etc., etc. and you will have some idea of what it is like up there on clinic days.

The girl students invited me up in the dissecting room this afternoon to see what nice work they were doing. So I lit a cigarette and paraded myself up to that Freshman's Paradise and criticized their work in most complimentary terms. I was glad enough to get out of there and have been feeling good ever since on account of my good fortune in not have to go there anymore.

Dec. 12, 1898:

I saw Randall Stoney this afternoon and he was looking very well indeed. He told me that he had had quite a hard time with his attack of pneumonia and had come very near dying. A woman attended him, so I suppose that is the reason that he managed to recover. She is Dr. Jacoby and is quite a noted physician in New York. Just wait until our two beauties graduate and then you will see what women can do.

It is my private opinion that Miss Viette will be such a warm member of the profession that she will dry up all of the rivers. I told her that she should be ashamed to flirt so openly with one of the students and what do you think she told me? She said that she had at first intended to flirt with me, but that as I did not seem inclined, she had given up the idea. She went on to say that she knew the reason so I said no more. Every time that she sees me on Monday she wishes to know if I have been to Summerville. I always say no. Is it right to tell her these stories? The only reason I do tell them is to keep her quiet. She has a very large mouth and she is inclined to do too much talking.

Taylor, a superior student, took part in the tradition of seniors helping freshmen:

Dec. 20, 1898:
There is a raffle of some kind at the college every day. The students get hard up at Christmas and they then proceed to raffle off pipes, watches,

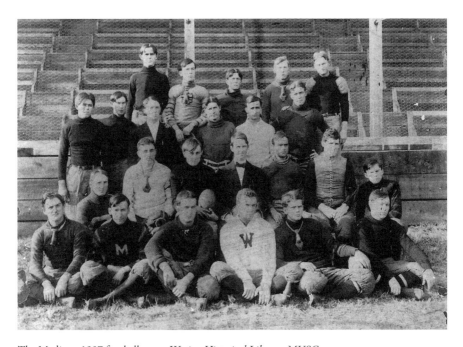

The Medicos, 1907 football team. *Waring Historical Library, MUSC.*

cuff buttons, bicycles, many things that they have and that people are willing to take a chance at. I suppose that you think the medical college is disintegrating into a den of thieves!

After Christmas I am to have a quiz class composed of three or four first year men, and I shall quiz them for an hour three times a week. There will be no fun in it, but as I am not doing it for fun, I do not mind that.

(Those composed young women who attended the Medical College with Taylor in 1898 both received their degrees in 1901 and went on to distinguished careers in medicine.)

Emilie Melanie Viett Rundlett, MD, was interviewed by William D. Sharpe, MD, in the 1950s. His biography of her was published in the *Journal of the South Carolina Medical Association*. He recalled their meeting:

On my first day on rotation through the contagious disease service at the Jersey City Medical Center late in the 1950's, I met an immensely dignified elderly lady physician who had a superficial—but *only* a superficial—resemblance to Aunt Pittipat Hamilton in *Gone With the Wind*. She didn't fool me—I'm half southern, and I know that these elderly ladies with their dotted Swiss dresses and cameo brooches are really made of barbed wire and harness leather. We became friends at first sight.

She recalled for Dr. Sharpe her years at the Medical College—including the perennial cadaver stunt:

We had the best men in town as teachers, and the Roper Hospital was wonderful! I really had no problems, though there were only two girls in our class. One of the students in anatomy cut part of his cadaver off—you can guess which part—and put it in the pocket of my pinafore. I knew that if I screamed, I was done, so I gritted my teeth, took it in my hand and marched right up to him. "Is this yours? You might need it."

Dr. Rundlett's career included being director of the Jersey City Medical Center Isolation Hospital, a fellow of the American College of Physicians and clinical professor of medicine at Seton Hall University; she also conducted a general practice, specializing in the diseases of women and children. Dr. Sharpe reported:

She became a distinguished and widely respected physician, and was in demand as a consultant in the care of the infections diseases of infants and children. An astute bedside clinician, she was a master of the small surgical techniques required for small patients, including endoctracheal intubation using her own set of sterling silver O'Dwyer's tubes...Emilie published one of the pioneer reports both of the diagnostic significance of cerebrospinal fluid glucose levels and of the efficacy of sulfadiazine in the treatment of meningococcal meningitis.

...She had a strong sense of persona. On one very memorable day, an intern resented the idea of an 80-year-old woman as an attending physician and, remarkably ill-bred, persisted in addressing her as "Mrs. Rundlett." The first time she heard this, Emilie was surprised; the second time, annoyed; but the third time! "I am old enough to be your grandmother, but I worked very hard to get to be called 'doctor,' and if you want to finish your internship here, do so."

The other woman in the first coed class, referred to by classmate Taylor as "a jewess," was Love Rosa Hirschmann Gantt. Dr. Gantt specialized in ophthalmology in Spartanburg and also had a long and active career in public health. In her president's address to the Medical Women's National Association in 1931, she remembered the progress of women in the medical profession:

It was in the early [eighteen] thirties, I think, that the first college, in that day scarcely more than a high school, was opened for the education of women. It was several years later in 1849 that the first woman was permitted to graduate in medicine. Some fifteen years later human slavery was banished, and it is less than a decade since women were recognized as the political equal of men and granted the right of suffrage.

It is in no spirit of levity, nor critical spirit that I call these facts to your attention, but simply that you may get some idea of how far we have advanced, in medicine, in education, in our social and political rights in the century that lies behind us.

(A few years after Viett and Hirschmann graduated, however, the presence of female students was "deemed undesirable," and women did not attend again until 1916; in 1921, the faculty granted them equal rights.)

CHAPTER 5

SYMPTOMS OF CHANGE
IN A NEW CENTURY

As medical education became serious business throughout the country—ever more focused on laboratory work, clinical practice, university hospital systems and reviews and ratings by the American Medical Association—the Medical College of the State of South Carolina determined to keep pace. Yet without an endowment or government support, financing new facilities, expensive equipment and competitive salaries posed a challenge. During the early years of the twentieth century, the college struggled and lost academic and professional ground to peer institutions. It barely managed to hold on until 1913, when the South Carolina legislature passed a bill that brought it into the state system of higher education.

By the time the college celebrated its centennial in 1924, female medical students had been welcomed back and the School of Nursing was a formal branch of the college. Pharmacy graduates had increased from a low of three in 1919 to twenty-seven in 1923. Mayor Thomas Stoney announced that Charleston would continue to strive to place its Medical College "on a parity with the very best that the United States has to offer." While recovery seemed assured, relapse also proved possible. The Great Depression would put the resiliency of students and doctors to the test.

RIGOR AND RELEASE FOR
TWENTIETH-CENTURY STUDENTS

Although the poverty of the state continued well after the war, the college determined to maintain rigorous graduation requirements. The catalogue of 1899–1900 announced a four-year program of study:

Requirements for Graduation in Medicine
The candidate must be twenty-one years of age, of good moral character, and have had a preliminary education satisfactory to the Faculty.

He must have attended four full courses of lectures, during four separate years, and have dissected during two sessions, in a Medical College recognized and approved by the Faculty, the last of which course of lectures must have been in this Institution.

He must have passed satisfactory examinations in all branches of the Curriculum.

He must have paid in full all College dues [with tuition and fees ranging from $100 in year 1 to $50 in year 4].

Medical College students of the early twentieth century became spirited about their institution and their experience, founding clubs, fraternity chapters and publications. Their new magazine, *Aesculapian*, provided a forum for both wit and scholarship:

Volume 1, Number 1, November 1909
We shall endeavor through the columns of "The Aesculapian" to draw the students nearer together, and thus promote a better college spirit; to keep the college constantly before the alumni and the academic students of the state and lastly, to stimulate a love for research work and the preparation of original articles by the students of the college...At the end of the College year a prize of ten dollars in gold will be given to the student who publishes in "The Aesculapian" the best original article on any medical or surgical subject.

Articles in the first edition included:

"The Anti-Tuberculosis Exhibition in Charleston"
"Some Deviations from The Normal in Human Structure"
"The Uses of Latin in Medicine"
"Medico-Pharmaceutical Relations"
"Syrup of Tar"

And some attempts at local humor:

Dr. Memminger to Soph. M: Have you any explanation for these numerous absences?
Mr. M: Yes, sir, I was homesick.

Landrum, after deciding to leave the College, told one of his friends that it was wrong for Dr. Wilson [the dean] not to let him enter with the Soph. Class after he had been here two months on "suspicion."

But the *Aesculapian* was short lived. In the final issue, October 1910, the editors included a plea to fellow students:

Dissecting Room Etiquette
At best, dissecting is not to the average student a very pleasant duty. Naturally he finds it more or less distasteful. One peculiar effect which it has upon some students is to bring to view the very worst elements of their natures. We realize that the student of science, in his search for truth, is supposed to consider the human body as a mere machine. However, we fail to see how coarse, boorish actions and unseemly practical jokes aid in the appreciation of anatomy. Secreting detached fingers, toes, ears, locks of hair and pieces of skin in a fellow student's pocket is a sorry exhibition of a depraved sense of humor, and, besides being disgusting, is liable to spread disease.

And a final lame joke:

Why is a porter on a Pullman car called doctor? Because he attends so many berths.

FOR NURSING STUDENTS, TOUGH DUTY CONTINUES

A second venture into nursing education, the Charleston Training School for Nurses, opened in 1895 with Medical College faculty as classroom instructors. Nurses were housed on the top floor of Riverside Infirmary and practiced nursing there, in City Hospital and in private duty. A hospital and training school for African American nurses was established in 1897 at 135 Cannon Street. City Hospital, partially demolished in 1904, was rebuilt as Roper Hospital with a new training school name—Roper Hospital Training School for Nurses—again sharing faculty and clinical work with the Medical College. However, the school would not officially come under the auspices of the Medical College until 1919.

Elizabeth (Bessie) Cork of Aiken, South Carolina, one of the first trainees at the new Roper Hospital, kept a daily diary of her required year of hospital duty—clearly a duty that was as exhausting as it was rewarding:

January 1, 1906. I am today at the Roper Hospital on the first day of her second existence. I have completed my examinations under the authorities of the Old City Hospital and am under obligations to serve twelve months in the new hospital before I shall receive my diploma...I am serving duty in White Female Ward with Miss Hoffman and have charge of Diet Kitchen.

January 8...Sent to Riverside. My Ward patients cried. I hated to leave, but like to work here.

13. Saturday. Have worked very hard this week and am to go on night duty tonight. Went out this afternoon with Miss Mary Sass to see the cruiser "Charleston." Received a letter from home.

14. Went on duty feeling fairly well. Was sick at eleven and came off duty.

15. Feel some better this morning. Dr. Rees came to see me. First professional visit I ever received from a Doctor. PM: Have been very sick all day. Someone sent me some flowers. Wish I knew who. Little things like that mean so much. Dr. Rees came again tonight. My head aches.

16. Feel better this morning, but Dr. Rees says I must remain in bed today. Received note from Dr. Jervey. He sent the flowers.

18. Worked, worked every minute. Went with Miss McLaurin to see her dress maker. Am going to bed with sore throat. Miss Alexander resigned her position to take a special case today.

27. An emergency operation for a bad case of appendicitis today added more to a hard day's work. Patient in No. 19 on my floor. Worked until 9 o'clock.

30. Mrs. Pedder was operated on today. I worked without a minute's rest till eight o'clock tonight.

Feb. 1. Had an hour to rest, but worked till nine o'clock.

Feb. 2. Worked all day again. Mr. and Mrs. McPherson gave me a cake in appreciation of my care...

Feb. 3 (Sat.). Admitted two new patients, Mr. W.C. Watts and little child Emily. Attended by Mrs. Watts, the young wife and mother. Both the sick ones have typhoid fever. It is a pleasure to have patients like these.

Sunday, 4th. Never have I worked so hard on any day before. But I think this is Sabbath, indeed, may the work of this day be blessed to His glory... Admitted Miss Cooner. Typhoid fever. There is a terrible epidemic of typhoid in the city (22 new cases today).

5: One cannot guess their own strengths till it is tested by a moral necessity. I have worked from seven a.m. to 10 p.m. without a minute's rest because upon my so doing the lives of sufferers depended...Sponged six times today.

6: Had an hour off. Went down the street to buy shoes. Sponged five times. Worked till 9 o'clock pm, 13 hours.

7. No time off, but got off duty tonight a little before eight...Mrs. Thrall gave me a splendid bottle of wine. I will drink it alone for my stomach's sake strictly. Lieut. Watts, my pet patient, is better today.

9. Lieut. Watts has been quite sick today. Sponged him five times. Had no hour off. Was on duty till 9:30 p.m. Mrs. Evison left with little kindly feeling for Riverside.

11. Went on duty as special nurse for Lieut. Watts. Very happy but it's very hard. Worked till eleven o'clock.

12. Patient very sick—worked till twelve. Sponged six times today. Tired.

13. Patient worse. Mother in law, Mrs. Scott, came today. Mrs. Watts is better. Worked till one o'clock.

14. Pt. very sick—worked till 2 a.m. But I love my patients therefore it is easy. His birthday. Is a shade better, I hope.

Feb. 17—March 12: All these following days were terrible battles and final despair and death...I never gave up...I am glad I have not tried to make a record of each day. The blank expresses more to my memory, for I had no other thought in those days, but to see that man get well and the efforts I made I cannot forget. If my own life had been asked in exchange for his recovery, it would have been freely given.

Margaret Isobel Wylie (Mrs. Eugene Jager), a 1913 graduate of the Roper Hospital Training School, also recalled strict rules and tight schedules. She was interviewed by Ruth Chamberlin, former dean of the School of Nursing, director of nursing at Roper Hospital and author of *The School of Nursing of the Medical College of South Carolina: Its Story* (reprinted by permission of the MUSC Alumni Association):

We had doctors' lectures at night in the basement of Roper Hospital—where the drug room was later. But our nursing procedures were taught by the head nurse or supervisor. She showed us one day, and we'd better do it the same way the next day. No textbooks either.

...With hands behind our backs we made rounds with the doctors. Only when the doctor went to the wash stand with its pitcher and bowl did we unclasp our hands. Then, we handed the doctor a linen towel. There was alcohol available too, if the doctor wanted to rinse his hands...

We got up at 6 a.m., had breakfast and full fifteen minutes of chapel before we got to the wards at 7 a.m. We worked 'til 7 p.m. with two hours off. We did get four hours off on Sundays. If we were on night duty, 7 p.m. to 7 a.m., we got no time off. Sleeping on duty would have been a penitentiary offense...

Each ward was divided with about 25 men in the first room and 20 women in the second. Two little rooms for very sick patients divided the men's and the women's sections. On our colored wards we called the men "Daddy" or "Uncle." The women answered to "Dah." Obstetrical patients were delivered in their beds in the women's surgical wards. There were screens, but there was no sound proofing.

Early twentieth-century limitations on medical knowledge and discovery made already difficult nursing assignments even more daunting for Nurse Wylie:

When I was in the colored medical ward, I had 17 typhoid patients at once and lost nine. We starved typhoid patients, I believe. They got only egg white and lemon juice for several days; then we added beef tea. We also gave the typhoids ice cold sponges to bring down their fever. Ice was brought to the wards by ice tongs, and we broke it up with an ice pick; no crushed ice or ice cubes were available.

Pneumonia offered a special province for us. Only nursing saved those patients. We breathed for them for five to nine days waiting for the crises. We wouldn't let them turn unassisted. Every effort was made to prevent any strain on the heart...We froze the tuberculosis patients. We put them on the porch with only one blanket in winter. Fresh air was the thing. But smallpox was sent to a contagious ward.

As the nursing school formally transitioned to become part of the Medical College in 1919, nursing directors continued as tough task masters with zero tolerance for deviation from diligence and obedience. Selections from a handwritten school ledger, 1915 to 1922, indicate that they minced no words in evaluating students:

- Nella A. (1919 graduate): Finished 3 year course, April 18, 1919. Had to serve 30 days extra for disloyalty—criticized operation surgeon before ward patients.
- Jane T. (1918 student): Entered upon probation. Not retained. Hard worker but too stupid—dense.

- Elsa P. (1918 student): Entered upon probation. Left of own accord. Objected to restrictions. Wished more freedom so as to attend dances, etc. Frivolous.
- Minnie W. (1919 student): She was allowed to leave at expiration of her two years as her work is not satisfactory and the school is better off without her presence.
- Alma K. (1919 student): This nurse did very poor work and was very impertinent. Left training after being reprimanded for slapping a little white girl on ward. Was married several days after leaving.
- Ursala D. (1919 student): Doing excellent practical work. Very conscientious and dependable. Class work excellent. Second honors in first year work.
- Ina S. (1921 student): Does very good practical work. Class work fair. Very popular with male sex and has been reprimanded and punished for breaking rules.
- Rose K. (1921 student): Has admitted violating Rule 5 Ethics of School Rules and Regulations by going to West Point with Dr. Kinny, an intern at Roper Hospital and a student at this Medical College.

While some students were being expelled for poor work or demeanor, others dropped out under the pressure of demanding studies and exhausting clinical work. Ledger entries for the student group of 1915 indicate that the training school was a very leaky ship indeed:

- Linda W.: Entered on probation. Resigned 1st day on colored ward, did not like it. Did good work, conscientious, but without aptitude.
- Lee P.: Entered on probation. Resigned. Complained of recurrence of eruption on hands.
- Ann S.: Deserted. Inefficient past record. Undesirable, not fit for the profession.
- Carrie F.: Entered on probation. Resigned. Good and obedient to rules. Refused to go on duty at Riverside.
- Mary S.: Deserted without reporting out. Not bright.
- Anna B.: Transferred on account of infected fingers.
- Thadie M.: Advised to resign. Incompetent. Not desirable material.
- Sarah B.: Dismissed for inefficiency and indiscretion.

Measuring Up Nationally?
Abraham Flexner Says "No"

The 1910 publication of *Medical Education in the Unites States and Canada*, written by Abraham Flexner, transformed medical education. Sponsored by the Carnegie Foundation for the Advancement of Teaching, Flexner spent three years visiting and analyzing medical schools throughout the country, and most of them he found hopelessly lacking—run for profit and without suitable academic entrance requirements, laboratories, clinical education or full-time faculty. The Medical College of the State of South Carolina, unfortunately, fell into the group of schools that Flexner suggested should be "wiped off the map":

> There yet remains for our consideration the third variety of school on the high school or equivalent basis, namely those described as basely mercenary. In point of equipment and teaching methods these schools are not substantially different from institutions on a still lower basis. Some of the latter institutions show, indeed, a better spirit: the University of Alabama, at Mobile, the College of Physicians and Surgeons and the School of Medicine, at Atlanta, the Medical College of the State of South Carolina, at Charleston, are not without traditions and a certain present dignity. Educationally, however, subject to certain exceptions to be specified from time to time, they may without violence be considered together; for limitations of one kind or another—now of equipment, now of intentions, again of both—make the effective teaching of any of the laboratory sciences frankly impossible.

Flexner's terse summary evaluation of the Medical College of South Carolina gave it a "Grade C" rating. Fortunately, the judgment happened when Robert Wilson, first honor graduate of the Medical College in 1892, was serving as dean. A bacteriologist, he joined the faculty in 1906 and had to persuade his colleagues of the germ theory of disease and that tuberculosis was not caused by holes in the lungs made by coughing. Named dean in 1908, a position he held for thirty-five years, Dr. Wilson understood that only state support could enable the Medical College to achieve a higher grade. He later recalled giving away the private medical school to the state:

> Having decided go to the legislature and persuade that body, if possible, to accept the college as a free-will gift, the next problem was how to approach

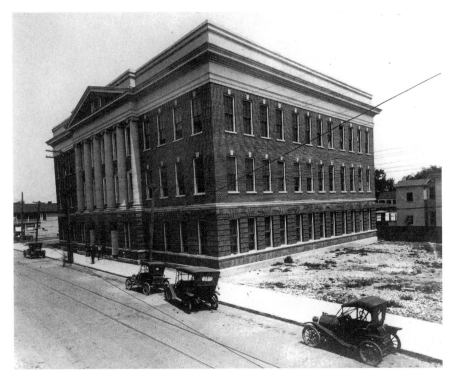

New Medical College building, 1914. *Waring Historical Library, MUSC.*

Governor Blease and secure his support without which the effort was foredoomed to failure. The chance discovery that for some unaccountable reason the Governor entertained a high opinion of me gave me the opportunity, and a suggestion of susceptibility to flattery afforded my cue.

Governor Coleman L. Blease, a notably flamboyant, explosive and shrewd politician, announced his support but recommended a change in control in his State of the State address, January 1913:

I recommend that an Act be passed making the Medical College at Charleston the Medical College of South Carolina, and making it a branch of the South Carolina University, and that you appropriate the sum of ten thousand dollars for the purpose of defraying the ordinary expenses of this institution. In my opinion it would add much to the educational system of the state.

Determined to keep the Medical College in Charleston and separate from the university, Dean Wilson wrote to every doctor in the state on behalf of his cause—except those in Columbia:

> We succeeded better than we had anticipated in keeping this information from the Columbia group. They heard of it accidentally at a county society meeting near Columbia only after the campaign had been set up, but it was too late then for them to organize the medical men of the state in opposition.

The legislation was passed on February 8, 1913, and just twelve days later, the Council on Medical Education of the American Medical Association changed the school's rating from C to B. Within weeks, the City of Charleston donated land, and Dean Wilson ushered in a new era with a successful campaign to raise $75,000 for the new Medical College building.

ONE STUDENT IN THE CLASS-B MEDICAL SCHOOL

Walter Haskell Harper, from Kingstree, South Carolina, attended the Medical College in the Class B years, graduating in 1916. He kept separate ledgers for each class, and though many pages are blank or filled with doodles, his notes reveal the diseases, treatments and assumptions of the day:

Pathology, notebook, 1914
On pneumonia:
   The age of the patient seems to be a factor. The two extremes of life seem to show a greater predisposition. Men are more subject than women because of more frequent exposure. Negroes are more susceptible than whites. Chinamen are very insusceptible.

Medicine notebook, 1914
Medicine Wednesday Oct. 14th 1914
Typhoid Fever:
   Typhoid Fever During the Third Week. The main danger in the third week of Typhoid fever is the increasing cardiac weakness, nervous weakness, complications, hemorrhages and perforations. During the fourth and fifth week, the patient's tongue clears up, abdominal symptoms are relieved, the fever gets lower, and the patient gets better. But the

patient may have secondary complications during the fourth and fifth week. And may get worse.

Dr. Jager, Medicine Jan. 6th 1915
Treatment of Scarlet Fever:
Isolate the patient. Have well ventilated room. Give buttermilk, ice-cream, milk, fruit juices, and plenty of water. Patient should be oiled every day with vasoline and ichthyol. Also should be sponged. May give ice or cold pack. Give nasal douches.

Doctoring Around the Globe

Early twentieth-century doctors, as well as Medical College students and alumni, took new strides toward globalizing medicine. Recent graduates began traveling abroad to contribute as missionaries in foreign clinics and researchers in disease control. John Wilson Bradley (class of 1896), for example, established modern medical facilities in China after arriving there with a Presbyterian mission in 1902. The next decade ushered in the Great War; and although most of the thirty-six faculty members who served in World War I were with medical and public health endeavors on the homefront, some saw active duty in Europe.

Another doctor with global intent, Theodore Hayne (class of 1927), undertook his internship in Panama, where his hospital rotations taught him a great deal about his career non-preferences, as reported in letters to his mother, "Fan" (Frances Thorn Hayne):

Ancon Hospital, Canal Zone, Nov. 25, 1927
Dear Fan:
Have been busy in the eye ear nose and throat department for the last week but don't think that I would prefer this branch of medicine for making a living, although it is said to be very remunerative. Have seen and assisted in tearing out a number of tonsils and adenoids but don't think the surgical technique is as good as that employed in the general surgical department...

The time is passing fast here because I'm so busy and interested in the work during the day and the interns find something to do almost every night. It's either a boat ride in the bay, a hike to the top of Ancon Hill, a dance at the Century club, or a swim in the large Balboa pool.

Not but more than seven more months when I shall have to begin making some money to pay back my numerous debts. Haven't decided exactly what to do but suppose that I shall take the first sure salaried job that will bring in the largest amount of money for a year or so.

    Love to all, Theodore

Hayne, who had spent some summers investigating malaria for the U.S. Public Health Service, soon returned to infectious disease research with a Rockefeller Foundation project studying yellow fever in Nigeria. He wrote home to advise his brother, Ike, about his studies at the Medical College and to report on his work:

West African Yellow Fever Commission, Lagos, Nigeria, November 5, 1928

Dear Ike:

    Your letter dated Sept. 29 arrived today and I sure was glad to hear that you had started at the Medical College. I wrote you a letter a few days ago, but had better answer this one while my enthusiasm is up...The work at the college will not be so hard if you study consistently every night and not save any work to be done during the week ends...Be sure to read your dissecting manual carefully each day before you go to class as it will make the work much easier. Also Dr. Philips [Professor William F.R. Phillips] has probably already told you that there are a certain number of pages to read each night in The Cunninghams, and it won't seem so much if you read the required amount each day. It pays a lot to talk a lot to your roommate about the work as discussing things with each other will help a lot to make you remember them...

    Your Brother, Theodore

During a three-month visit home to Congaree, South Carolina, in early 1930, Hayne married Roselle Hundley. Due to yellow fever, bubonic plague and other prevalent diseases in Nigeria, he returned alone to Africa to complete his tour with the Rockefeller Foundation project, reporting to his brother:

June 22, 1930

Dear Ike

    Your long letter was received on the last mail and I know that now you are out of the fog and have completed the first year of medicine at the medical college...

    Besides maintaining all of the strains of yellow fever virus in the monkeys and mosquitoes here, I have to do a lot of outside work trying to study something of the life habits and relative importance of the eight or nine mosquitoes other than the aedes aegypti that have been shown in the laboratory to transmit the disease.

...The problem of Yellow Fever in West Africa seems less and less feasible as we go along. I knew it was going to take a long time and a lot of money but thought that the fact of our doing some work here might add something to our knowledge of its endemicity...

...I shall probably get my tour here shortened from eighteen months. I certainly hope so.

Your brother, Theodore

In July 1930, Theodore Hayne contracted yellow fever in Nigeria. He died four days later. In 1931, a new vaccine was developed that proved effective in protecting against the disease.

SOME THINGS DON'T CHANGE:
ANATOMY OF A PROFESSOR

Dr. William Cyril O'Driscoll taught anatomy to first-year students for fifty-three years. A graduate of the Medical College in 1905, O'Driscoll joined the faculty in 1908 and became a beloved and charismatic teacher. He made his own visual aids: intricate and colorful drawings of organs, models of body parts constructed from scraps of metal—sometimes from the folds of his lab coat. Able to write with either hand and backward and forward, he was famous for his demonstrations, but perhaps more famous for his retorts.

To the student who smoked a cigarette during the first lecture:

Dammit, man, you've got so much gall, if your gallbladder burst, you'd drown.

For students coming to his office, a large sign:

This is a busy office. Please limit yourself to three minutes.

To any women in his class:

Always an advocate of Women's Suffrage. And by God, I'm here to see them suffer.

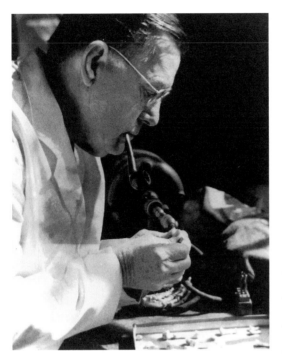

Left: Dr. O'Driscoll wiring the bones of a hand. *Waring Historical Library, MUSC.*

Below: Drawing of an ear by Dr. O'Driscoll. *Waring Historical Library, MUSC.*

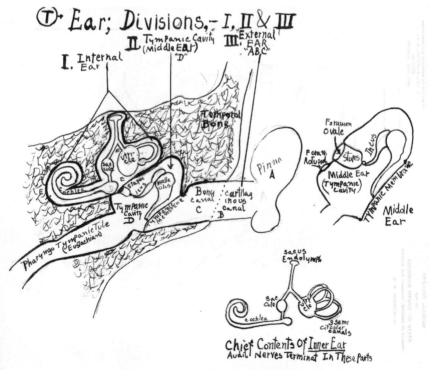

To students struggling to learn anatomy:

Find it on your body!
To a student who asked "doc" for some help:

You can call me Mister, you can call me Professor, you can call me Junior, or you can call me Doctor. But don't you ever "doc" me again.

To the student who didn't want to return to the dissecting laboratory on Sunday:

Son, you know the story in the Bible of the man whose ass fell into the ditch on the Sabbath and Jesus said the ass could be pulled from the ditch on the Sabbath without violating the laws of God? Well, son, your ass is in the ditch.

No Certain Treatment
for the Great Depression

Medical education during the Depression years combined academic challenges with financial ones. The experiences of Dr. Alton G. Brown Sr. (class of 1939), as well as his difficulties and sacrifices, are revealed in his unpublished manuscript, *Memoirs of a Retired Surgeon and War Diaries*:

I finished my college career [University of South Carolina] in May, 1933, which was the very depth of the depression. Many, many people were committing suicide. It was a difficult time to search for work. The government had organized the Civilian Conservation Corps as an emergency organization to help young people who were coming out of school and who were out of work.

After professors at the university allowed students to miss final exams and receive diplomas by mail, Brown was sent to the CCC camp in Ridgeland, South Carolina:

Our camp was well-organized. Since I was a pre-med student, I worked in the infirmary. It was a relatively easy job, but I spent more time taking a first aid kit out to the woods and voluntarily digging stumps, cutting trees, cleaning swamps, and fighting fires than sitting in the infirmary. There were two of us in the infirmary, and at least every couple of days, the army doctor would come out and check patients and take care of minor surgery. We would take care of the minor accidents and sick calls for the other part of the time. Our pay was $30 a month, and I believe $25 was sent home. I am sure it was greatly needed in many of the homes, but since our home was mostly self-sufficient, my father kept my money in a separate account for me to use to go to medical school.

...During the following summer, I was accepted for medical school at the Medical College of South Carolina in Charleston. I took a trip down for an interview with Dr. Cy O'Driscoll. He was in the Anatomy Department and was head of admissions. He was a great old fellow. Since my brother J.J. had not yet married, he agreed to send me $50 a month to help me do this even though I had a little money saved...

I managed to make enough in the summer to reregister for classes in the fall. With the $50 loan each month from my brother J.J., I managed to scrape through another year of school. During my sophomore year I worked in Dr. Lassick's [probably Dr. Arthur M. Lassek] laboratory and was also prosector. In other words, I dissected a cadaver a week ahead of time for the professor to use as an illustration for the freshman.

Each year in school was a little different from the other. The first year is probably the hardest because there is not much practical work. As we went further into our study, we began to get physical diagnosis, actually examined patients, and went to the hospital with the professors. Later, we would even see our own patients and do lab work as our education progressed. The practice hospital for the medical students was the old Roper Hospital; it was the hospital that took care of all the charity work in Charleston. It was so crowded that frequently large wards had so many beds that you could not get between the beds to examine patients. We would have to pull the bed out to examine them. A great number of beds were occupied by patients with osteomyelitis and great weeping wounds and sores. We had no antibiotics at that time, so the infected bone was saucerized or curetted out and packed open to let heal. Many of the wounds recurred and spread over the body. From a practical viewpoint, I learned a great deal during my last two years.

...As interns, we were expected to work up the new patients to do their laboratory work, to write up their histories and physicals, and most of the time to assist the surgeons in surgery. How we worked all that in plus our studies and work at Roper Hospital I don't really know...

...I would start out each fall weighing about 170 pounds and in excellent shape, but by the end of the year I would weigh about 130 pounds due to all my hard work and studying.

All that, and a polio epidemic too:

Nellie Claire Sanders and I were united in marriage at 8:00, the morning of June 2, which was the morning following my graduation from the medical college. There had been a polio epidemic during the last part of my senior year. Thus, crowds had been limited to 50 or less so we did not plan a graduation ceremony. At the last minute they let us have a graduation ceremony in a little theater.

We could only invite the immediate family, but on such short notice, it was too late for me to invite any of my family. It so happened that I led my class most of my four years in medical school. With a lot of hard work and studying I had been making straight A's. and there was a race between Francis Cole and me as to who might be first honor student. On graduation night they announced that I was first honor student.

(Dr. Brown's high marks earned him an internship at Cincinnati General Hospital, one of the most competitive in the country. Francis Hammond Cole eventually became a professor of surgery at the University of Tennessee.)

Dr. H. Rawling Pratt-Thomas (class of 1938), who would eventually serve as president of the Medical College (1962–64), also kept a frantic pace of part-time work, studies and clinical duties in order to struggle through a medical education during the Great Depression. In his 2002 memoir, *From Yorkshire Pudding to Hominy Grits: Exhumation of a Pathologist's Life*, he recalled clearly and candidly the life of a medical student during his college years:

Medical schooling during the 1930s was conducted in an atmosphere of terror. The various committees and assorted deans that today overlook a student's progress and well-being were non-existent. The most common phrase drummed into our ears by upper classmen was "You're going to flunk!". The attitude of the faculty was that the students were interlopers and were here only at the sufferance of the faculty, who were going to do everything possible to prevent intrusion into their select fraternity.

Well before "ratemyprofessor.com," student assessments of faculty circulated freely and frequently, according to Pratt-Thomas:

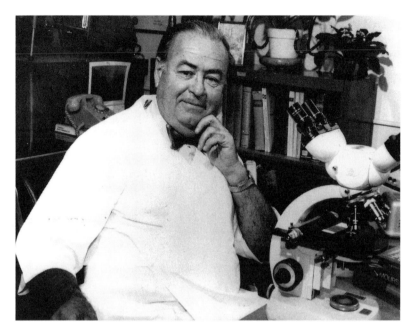

Dr. H. Rawling Pratt-Thomas, professor, dean and president of the Medical College of South Carolina, 1962–64. *Waring Historical Library, MUSC.*

Robert Spann Cathcart, "The Colonel," Chairman and Director of the Department of Surgery, was arbitrary and dictatorial. He was dubbed "Great God Almighty" by the students…He would occasionally call to a student "young man, come here. What is your name?" This was tantamount to disaster as the legend had developed that should you be so summoned by Dr. Cathcart, you would flunk at least Surgery and probably in totality…

Surgeon Dr. William Prioleau affectionately became known as the "thyroid thief" because of his proclivity for thyroidectomy. Dr. Prioleau also made a fetish of sterile surgical technique…[His] influence is still with me today…my wife inquires, "Why are you washing your arms?" I would reply "because Dr. Prioleau taught me to do it this way."

The professors having the greatest impact on the incoming medical student in any School of Medicine are always the professors of Anatomy. My class was no exception. We were greeted by two memorable and vividly contrasting personalities, Arthur Marvel Lassek and William Cyril O'Driscoll. The former, young, handsome, restrained, taciturn, cold. The latter older, voluble, gregarious, earthy…Lassek was, in the vernacular, a cold fish. We quickly dubbed him "The Great Stone Face."…

Dr. O'Driscoll was probably the most outstanding professional character that I have ever known…

Pathology was taught by Kenneth Merrill Lynch…a Texan who became the first full time professor of pathology as well as the first full time faculty member of the Medical College of the State of South Carolina in the summer of 1913. He was an excellent teacher and a friend of the medical students…

John van de Erve, "the Dutchman," was Chairman of the Department of Physiology…Of all the professors to confront the medical student, he inspired the greatest dread. The reason for this terror was Dr. van de Erve's well-established proclivity for failing the majority of his class. He struck them down with impunity, to such an extent that the faculty had to reason with him, in order to avoid self-liquidation—no medical students to teach.

Pratt-Thomas also recalled problematic facilities:

My clinical experience took place in Roper II. This hospital has been completed in February 1906 and functioned as the teaching hospital for the Medical College of the State of South Carolina for fifty years. Roper II was the Hospital of the Four Senses, only taste being lacking…

Sounds subtle and blatant permeated one's surrounding, many subliminal, others raucous. The slushing of the steampipes, the clamorous, knocking radiators in winter, the somnolent drone of the electric fans, thrown out of key by the buzzing flies in summer, the cries from those in pain, or of someone suddenly bereaved…Bats dodging the roentgen rays in the radiology department and in turn, being dodged by scrambling patients and technicians; the silent repulsive sentries of the night, gray-brown shadows of the rats in the emergency entrance, the parking lot beyond, or even daring the corridors.

CHAPTER 6

THE GREATEST GENERATION

The Great War, in spite of its billing, was not the war to end all wars. Another one was brewing. Graduates of the Medical College would witness the unimaginable carnage firsthand as they risked—and sometimes lost—their lives in trying to alleviate the suffering on the many fronts of World War II. Years later, in the 1990s, Dr. Laurie Brown (class of 1953), navy yeoman during the war and professor and chairman of anesthesiology, solicited World War II reminiscences from twenty-eight South Carolina physicians who had been in active service. Some sent him their war diaries, some sent unpublished manuscripts, some wrote letters and some talked to him or into tape recorders.

THE ARMY RECRUITS DOCTORS

Dr. Sol Neidich of Beaufort (class of 1937) remembered:

> In 1937, during my senior year at the Medical College of S.C., a team of high ranking U.S. Army Medical Corp Officers visited our school to encourage service in Military Medicine and offered a 1st Lieut. Commission upon graduation, in the Reserve Corps. As a result of this invitation, half of our class of 42 Seniors joined. Many were in private practice in small towns throughout South Carolina prior to Dec. 1941 and were declared essential.

Then came the trauma of Pearl Harbor. Dr. Thomas Marion Davis (class of 1943), later general surgeon, from Manning, South Carolina, recalled:

> My daddy was a clerk in a store and he didn't have any money. And, so, I was just about, really, getting right panicky. And, I was studying just before this, I

was studying up in the Histology Lab on Sunday morning and had the radio going and we were looking in microscopes giving each other histology practicals and they interrupted the radio program to say that the Japanese Navy had bombed Pearl Harbor (I didn't know where Pearl Harbor was). And then it was chaos and then, of course, President Roosevelt declared war on the Japanese and not long after that, the Medical College was taken over by the military. And, we were given the option of either joining the V-12 program, which was a Navy program, or the ASTP [Army Specialized Training Program] which was an Army program. (There were two girls in my class—they didn't join anything.) There were two boys in our class who refused to join. But everybody else in my class either wore a PFC Army uniform or a Navy midshipman's uniform.

For Davis, always out of money, the war was good news—at first:

I chose the Navy. And they paid us $150 a month, they furnished us the uniforms, a uniform allowance, they bought our books, they paid our tuition. And we were home free. That was a wonderful thing. Wonderful thing for me. Of course, in return, when I got through interning I joined the Navy and served and went overseas and was attached to the 1st Marine Division in the Pacific and on up to Okinawa as a Battalion Surgeon which means you hit the beach with the Marines. So I paid them back.

WAR IN THE PACIFIC

Davis's internship in Columbia was reduced to nine months because of the war. Then he was shipped out to Okinawa. He remembered treating soldiers in battle:

We had a lot of blood. We used a lot of blood. And they, it seemed to me like they had it packed in dry ice and they would bring it up (and we were on the front lines—sometimes in front of the front lines!) and we would give them blood transfusions. We did not have a hospital. We would see these men on the ground behind a huge rock, behind trees, and we would give the blood and plasma, we used a lot of plasma and did the best we could—put on splints and so forth and put them on a jeep ambulance and sent them down the mountain and to a tent hospital which was back in the rear about ten miles. But we were right up in the front. And we used a lot of sulpha drugs and we didn't do any fancy repairing up there. We put clamps, we put hemastats on bleeders. It wasn't sterile. We did not have any rubber gloves. We washed our hands and did the best we could, but we were right out there in the open, in the woods with a helmet on and dungarees, I wore dungarees.

...They brought a Captain in and he was wounded, a superficial wound, and he was exhausted and he hadn't had any sleep in about four days and four nights, he was wet and he was muddy, and I made him drink a cup of coffee. I said I'm giving you an order, you've got to stay here tonight and sleep...The next morning he felt better, he was just combat fatigued. So he was about my size, so I gave him a set of clean underwear and I gave him my set of clean dungarees and they had my name stenciled on the back. Lt. T.M. Davis, USNR...so the next day I was working on casualties, I heard two of the men that they brought in say, "We sure are sorry about Lt. Jeff Davis," (they called me Jeff Davis because I was a southerner) I said, "What about him?" They said, "He got killed up on the airport last night." And, of course, it was the poor fellow I had given my jeans to.

Dr. Davis remembered classmates lost in battle:

In fact, several boys that I knew were killed over there. Fellow named "Boobie" Nelson [perhaps J.D. Nelson, class of 1936] was at Iwo Jima, right across the water from us; he was in the army. He was from North, S.C. He was an intern a year ahead of me. He was killed over there. And John Cathcart [class of 1927] was in the Army and killed in the Philippines by a sniper. He was tending to a man and the sniper shot him and they put him on a stretcher, started to evacuate him and the sniper shot him down and he killed him. He was from Winnsboro, S.C.

THE WAR IN EUROPE

Dr. Alton G. Brown Sr. (class of 1939) had entered the army before Pearl Harbor. He was first sent to California for training, where he encountered the legendary General Patton. Dr. Brown followed Patton's entire European campaign and wrote about it in his unpublished journal, *Memoirs of a Retired Surgeon and War Diaries*:

Indio, California
11th Evacuation Hospital Desert Training Center
May 10, 1942

Speaking of General Patton, commonly known everywhere as "Old Blood and Guts," he talked to us again yesterday. All officers and men lined up and marched two and a half miles in the dust and sun and gathered in an assembly point. After waiting an hour until the proper time, he arrived…He talked for half an hour telling of the advantages of going without food for long periods of time. Patton's chief asset is his vulgarity and profanity. He loves to call the enemy filthy names and can also call his own men the same at times.

He soon learned that the army's medical equipment was out of date:

June 29, 1942

We are supposed to have 47 officers at war strength. That is the number they had in 1918 and I understand that the army hasn't developed or advanced an inch in some ways since then. With an entirely new type war and new developments in medicine, we are to be an evacuation hospital with the same type equipment that an Evacuation Hospital had in 1918. In fact, lots of the equipment hasn't been unpacked since it was put up for the last war.

Aboard the former ocean liner *Monterey*, Dr. Brown was part of a convoy headed for Africa:

Aboard Ship
November 3, 1942

After breakfast, I went on deck for the first time and it was a sight to behold. We were in a smooth sea, out of sight of land and one of a large convoy. There are probably 35–40 ships in the convoy, including transports, freighters, tankers, aircraft carriers, battle ships, cruisers, and destroyers. It was a beautiful sight with seaplanes flying around the convoy and several blimps cruising around.

November 11, 1942

Today is Armistice Day, that day when years ago all the world rejoiced at the ending of murder and butchery. Today, even a worse war is in full blast with many fields covered with blood, thousands dying and millions more innocent young men who will die before another armistice.

Dr. Brown saw those wounded and dying up close as he worked twelve-hour shifts in an evacuation hospital in Tunisia:

April 11, 1943

We are still bivouacking a few miles from Constantine. Many planes roar overhead. All day transport planes have been going back and forth across our area. It is hard to think of these ambulance planes, each probably loaded with 13 seriously wounded, going back to hospitals.

April 28, 1943

German prisoners talk much more than I expected and give me hope. One said people no longer have any heart for war. Ten days ago, he was on the Russian front—flown here.

Dr. Brown followed the entire European campaign:

Licata, Sicily

July 17, 1943

It is 8 p.m., and I just finished 12 hours at the operating table. We have a real war on now...Last night our forces near here captured Agrigento. Beginning at dark, casualties came in all night, and the team was quite busy. Italians would gladly surrender, but the Germans won't let them.

July 19, 1943

We had a few Germans in last night and many are coming in today also. They are just ordinary humans who are frightened, hurting and worried with pictures of wives and cute children in their pockets. Last night, side by side was a German and an American soldier. I worked on both. I couldn't help but feel how idiotic war is. It is just missed humans.

Sometimes field hospitals were more dangerous than battlefields:

Anzio Beachhead

April 29, 1944

Last night was a noisy one...At its height, it was terrific, and then the planes would dive over our area, and in spite of the din of guns, they could be heard screaming down straight at the hospital...When the planes come low everything opens up and flak falls everywhere...Poor patients in the wards feel helpless as there is no shelter over their heads, and up front they have trouble getting men to go to the hospital unless they are very sick or badly wounded. They feel safer in a foxhole. Last night many were under their beds, and begging for shovels to dig foxholes with…A fellow has been known to come to the hospital for medical causes and go out with a purple heart and two clusters for wounds received in the hospital…

Anzio, Italy
June 6, 1944
 ALLIES INVADED FRANCE TODAY…We know few details but know there are thousands of ships, divisions of paratroopers, and thousands of planes.

Dr. Brown followed the invasion to France and, at last, to Germany:

Off Coast of France
August 15, 1944
 …At present the cruisers, destroyers and battleships are rolling in a heavy barrage, shaking the air around us…Great tongues of flame would leap out from their large guns, followed by a terrific roar and air blast. To join this many hundred heavy and medium bombers came over from various directions.

Dayon, France
October 22, 1944
 The push is apparently on and spreading along this whole front. We ran out of blood about noon and expected the bank to bring some by. When the truck arrived, they were also out of blood.

Gollheim, Germany
March 26, 1945
 There used to be a time when our hospital moved in two trips with our trucks as we are supposed to, but now we have accumulated so much that 4 long trips will be necessary…The French people were sorry to see us go.

In May 1945, just a week before victory in Europe, Dr. Brown gave typhus shots to two war correspondents, one from CBS and one from the London *Daily News*. They invited him along on their assignment:

Dillingen, Germany
May 3, 1945
 …We got to Dachau at about noon. That is the most famous of Germany's concentration camps. Dachau itself is a nice pretty little town

practically undamaged by war. The first signs of anything out of the ordinary are scenes on railroad tracks leading into the town and camp. A long train, some 59 cars long, stands on the track, mostly boxcars, low and high, and most of these are still partially filled with human bodies. They lie grotesquely on the boxcar floors. Some died trying to crawl out while others were outside the cars. The odor would be very bad except for the cold weather. Near the cars and along the roads are bodies of a dozen or so German S.S. men, lying where they fell.

We went on into the camp area, a mile or so from the town proper, perhaps. Inside a large gateway are beautiful administrative buildings, and along the edges of the big estate are magnificent villas and dwellings of the commandants and big shots. In the administrative buildings, the Americans have taken over and have offices of various kinds running the camp and trying to straighten out a horrible mess. The 116th Evac has taken over one building setting up a hospital...I am very glad we didn't draw that job for many reasons...

Our first trip was to the incinerator buildings. This building composed of several large rooms and an attached building or two is a chamber of horrors. At one end is a huge pile of clothes of all types which were taken from the victims. Inside the main doorway is the furnace room, and here are some five or six furnaces large enough to accommodate several bodies each at a time. In the large room to the right, there are piled, yes, piled in great heaps, twisted and distorted, clothed, partly clothed and unclothed, literally thousands of human bodies, mostly emaciated wrecks. Apparently, most mainly died of starvation, plus the final gas treatment...Over the gas chamber door is a sign in German that says "Shower Room." The victims are herded in here, gassed, and then dumped into the storage rooms until they are burned...

...At present, prisoners are being screened by authorities, and some are being released to start the journey to their homes by foot and carrying their belongings. This seems horrible, but they were very happy. Many will die. Others are probably warped mentally and their lives are ruined...

Many correspondents think the next few days will end it all. I am quite tired and will go to bed, but I will likely dream of depraved mankind and his actions.

VICTORY IN EUROPE

Dr. Brown's war ended with victories, medals and a practical assessment:

Dillingen, Germany
May 8, 1945
...I have just heard Prime Minister Churchill officially announce the end of the war in Europe. Papers were signed yesterday and the cease fire order was given, but officially all ends tonight at one minute after midnight. Some fellows are still hard at work occupying areas, taking prisoners, some E.G. troops are still fighting, and some hospitals are probably still busy. Many lie wounded in hospitals and some of these will not live to get home...

Dillingen, Germany
May 19, 1945
Last night's formation was for presentation of Bronze Stars to Major Alton Brown and Sgt. Hopkins. My citation stated that I had worked long hours in surgery of my own volition, besides the job of running the lab. It is nice to get an award, but I feel a bit embarrassed as surgery was a break for me.

Processed for separation at Fort Bragg, North Carolina, in August 1945, Alton Brown summed up his war experience:

The medics there were pretty upset to see other medics get out (though they had not been in long or been overseas). One sarcastically asked how I did it. I said "Oh it's easy. Just give 4½ years service, 33 months of combat service, 7 campaign stars, a decoration, and 144 points." They made no more comments.

VICTORY IN JAPAN

The war was not over in the Pacific or for Harold E. Jervey, desperately hoping to be released in time to enter the Medical College in the fall of 1945. Jervey had spent four years as a navy lieutenant in the Pacific, and at the end of the war was aboard a ship that had captured the Japanese vessel *Tachibana Maru* carrying 1,538 armed combat troops. His account, "No Bands Played," was never published but is part of Dr. Laurie Brown's collection of reminiscences:

Monday 6 August 1945

Arriving at the ship [in Morotai Harbor] Tuesday morning 7 August we looked like a new crew. What a difference food, rest, fresh uniforms and a shave made. Photographers and reporters from national wire services and major magazines such as Life and Time were everywhere. This was an unprecedented story! The capture of a ship with the largest number [1,538] of able bodied Japanese troops ever taken prisoner during the war with the smallest number [80] of men. All of this without a single casualty. The American public and the world needed to know; at once!

It didn't happen that way. The headlines and lead stories screamed, "World's First Atomic bomb Dropped on Hiroshima." The capture of the Tachibana Maru was relegated to a supporting role…At 0805 Wednesday 15 August the Charrette signaled: "President Truman has declared the war is officially over."…In Japan a new government under Prince Toshihiko Higahikuni was being formed. More importantly mail arrived! My father's letter was the big news. I let out a yell.

"Just listen to this fellers. My place in the freshman class at medical school is being held. The Dean has told my father, It's mine whenever I arrive. Ain't that something?"

Ken Miller didn't' share my enthusiasm and remarked, "You must be nuts! School is starting September 4th. It's the 17th of August. It'll take a miracle for you to get there. Even if you do, you're four years away from college subjects. I don't see how you're going to make it."

Lieutenant Jervey flew to Pearl Harbor and waited to be released, but instead received a new command aboard the *President Hayes* in Tokyo:

I knew medical college was out for now and perhaps forever. I drowned my sorrows at the bar ranting and raving about the callous, stupid asses running the Navy…I explained to Kirven [senior officer of the day] if my orders weren't changed I would have to give up the goal of medicine as a career.

"I'm on your side Lieutenant," a pleasant voice said. "Get down here the first thing in the morning and I'll take care of your orders."

I just uttered. "Thanks."

The orders came through and so did the Medical College:

I'm still in a whirl. Got a letter from my father saying they were definitely expecting me for this class at Med School. Just think! Two days ago I had given that up. Today everything is going according to plan. It's not such a bad world, is it?

Another doctor viewed another kind of carnage. Dr. Frederic MacNaughton Ball graduated from the Medical College in the accelerated class of 1943 and saw active duty in the Medical Corps of the United States Navy Reserve aboard ships in the Pacific and naval hospitals in the United States. He wrote to his parents from Japan:

October 26 1945: "THE TRIP TO THE MODERN POMPEII"
Yesterday I saw Hiroshima. We left the ship at 8:30 and took off in the jeep from Hiro in the direction of Kure and Hiroshima...Beyond Kure the paved highway ran along the water's edge—a part of the inland sea and an extension of Hiroshima Wan...Finally we got to the MP stop outside Hiroshima where we had to show our permit to enter the city's ruins. We had gotten a pass the day before from Kure on the excuse that we were going in on "medical research." The bomb had exploded just over the residential and business district of the city and what wasn't melted or pulverized by the terrific heat and pressure was burned by the later fires...

...We wandered around and about taking pictures and picking up bits of china and fused glass for souvenirs. The foundations of houses were easy to make out but all wall, roofs and floors were collapsed flat or burned away—only china withstood the heat at all—bedsteads, stoves, parts of sewing machines, glassware automobiles, bicycles and so forth were twisted and melted. Metal scaffold type towers built for carrying high-tension power lines through the city were bent over at the base, leaning away from the center of the blast. The city had been cleaned of bodies and there was no overpowering odor of decay. Altho the smell of open sewers was not appreciated. I walked in the ruins of one house in which the remains of the tiled kitchen and bath were still distinguishable. Wine bottles still stood under the sink and food (burned black) still stood in little dishes in the tiled oven. The general impression of the whole place was that of a populous city suddenly and instantly knocked down by a blast of tremendous heat.

The Japs are beaten and know it but they do not grovel in defeat. If I had to spend any more time in the Pacific I couldn't do better than in Japan—but I hope I'm coming home soon.

To get back to Hiroshima—we have had several arguments on the justification of snuffing out 100,000 lives in a few seconds in an area in which military installations were at a minimum...I believe the only possible justification rests in the fact that war in the future will literally wipe out urban civilization and on the possibility that this fact will sober people when they get worked up next time. It is only justified if it ends wars. Maybe it did cause the Japs to quit sooner but who can prove that they wouldn't have quit short of invasion anyway?

I have the news that we will be bringing troops to the west coast soon. This is definite. Maybe I'll be home for Christmas!

All my love and God bless you both—

Your son Mac.

At Last, the Veterans Come Home

Those who returned to the Medical College found mixed reactions from the faculty. Dr. Thomas Marion Davis received his orders to return in May 1946 and then performed physicals on those being discharged at the Sixth Naval District Hospital. He recalled:

So I didn't know when I was going to get out. So I went down to the Medical College and talked to some friends and went by to see Dr. L.A. Wilson, to see about getting a residency in OB/GYN he had promised me before the war. Or during the war when I was finishing medical school...he could be a rather acid man—chain smoked—always had a Pall Mall in his hand—and so I walked in there and I had on a Marine uniform, First Division Patch on it and all, and he said, where did you get that monkey suit?

I said, "Well, I'm in First Marine Division."

He said, "I hate Marines." And I just kind of let that slide.

I said, "What I came by to see you wasn't to discuss the Marine Corps, but to see how soon I can start a residency in OB/GYN."

He said, "Well, you're not going to get a residency in OB/GYN."

I said, "Sir?"

He said, "You're not going to get a residency in OB/GYN. I'm looking out for fellows who stayed here during the war and looked out for me. You guys who got flag happy and left here, as far as I'm concerned are out in the cold."...

I couldn't believe how I felt. But I walked across the street to see Dr. Lynch who was the Dean of the Medical School. And he was very cordial. A wonderful personality. We chatted and I brought him up to date on what I was doing. "What are your plans, he asked." I said, "Well, I'd like to have a residency in OB/GYN but Dr. Wilson said I didn't have a cut dog's chance of getting one here"...He laughed and said "Well, I'll tell you why said that, because I've known him for a long time. In World War I a marine took the girl he was engaged to and married her. He doesn't like you people."

Dr. Horace Smithy, an associate professor of surgery, was not amused by Dr. Wilson's revenge. He arranged a surgical residency for Dr. Davis:

So I went to work at the Roper Hospital as a first year Surgical Resident on the first of July in the old Roper Hospital; It had hot and cold running roaches and hot and cold running rats...But I enjoyed my time down there. Made lots of friends. Dr. Smithy, he was very temperamental, he was a very smart man, way ahead of his time. He had a bad heart problem himself. It was aortic stenosis and he eventually died of it. He was 37. [actually 34] Died of heart failure at 37. So I didn't get to work with him very long.

Dr. Horace Gilbert Smithy Jr. devised a new operating technique and cutting instrument to remove scar tissue in heart valves caused by rheumatic fever, a disease he too had suffered from. His successful operation on Betty Lee Woolrich received national attention months before his own death in 1948.

Dr. Alton G. Brown came back to Charleston and the Medical College, still strapped for cash:

16 King Street
Charleston S.C.
June 30, 1946
...Tomorrow morning I take over the duties as Chief Resident at Roper Hospital for a year, and Chief Surgical Resident as well as Teaching Fellow in Surgery at the Medical College and believe I will have a wonderful year's experience...

It took me and most other veterans six more months to get anything out of the Veterans Administration in the way of aid under the G.I. Bill. At last I am getting a monthly check of $90. It is a wonderful help and I also have $500 a year with the college for purchase of books and instruments, etc. and have gotten about three hundred dollars worth. Even with $250 pay, $90 a month from Vet. Adm I can't begin to get by.

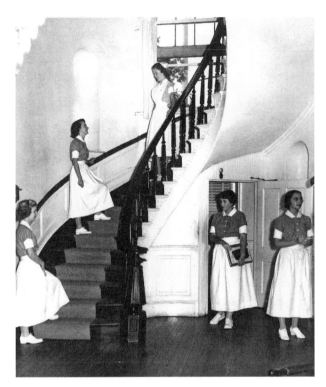

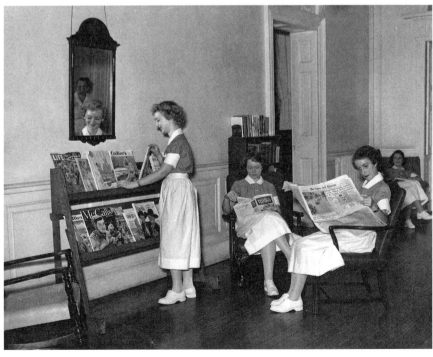

Left: Nursing students in residence hall, 1949. *Courtesy of College of Nursing, MUSC.*

Below: Off-duty nurses, 1948. *Courtesy of College of Nursing, MUSC.*

Harold E. Jervey Jr., sailing home on *Monssen DD798* in September 1945, knew that he was late:

> This damn ship just doesn't move fast enough. School started on 4 September. The closer I get to my arrival the less certain I am of my decision. I don't really know if I'll like medicine. What if I bust out? I made this decision early in the war.

He arrived at the Charleston Navy Yard on October 5, 1945, and went right to school:

> I was pleased to learn I had been promoted to Lt Cmdr. Momentarily I thought: Maybe I ought to stay in. I might make Admiral and run the Navy. That was quickly dismissed and with uniform on I went downtown and reported in to my new station: Medical College of S.C. At the registrar's office I filled in forms. "Do you want to start right now?" he asked.
>
> "You betcha," I replied.
>
> "I'll show you to your class. You'll be interested in meeting your classmates and they you."
>
> I was apprehensive when I was introduced to Dr. Cy O'Driscoll Professor of Anatomy. He did nothing to allay my fears. "Where have you been? This class has been going for five weeks. We've finished one dissection and are almost through the second."
>
> I knew I had made a big mistake. The feeling changed when he put his arm about my shoulder and with a smile said, "Let's meet your classmates."
>
> Entering the door I was overpowered with the stench of formaldehyde and grotesque looking cadavers. Why had I thought I wanted to study medicine? This was the war all over again and a stinking one at that.
>
> O'Driscoll said with his arm still around me, "This is Lt. Cmdr. Harold Jervey your long awaited classmate. Give him a big welcome."
>
> I stared at the ghoulish creatures nonchalantly chewing gum and fingering cadaverous flesh. They looked at me and my ribbons as though I were an alien from outer space. Would this be another war on another ocean with another ship?

(Dr. Jervey married Lil, graduated from the Medical College in 1949, had seven children and practiced for many years in Columbia, South Carolina.)

CHAPTER 7

SYSTEMIC GROWTH AND DEVELOPMENT

D r. Kenneth Lynch, who had become the first full-time faculty member of the Medical College in 1913, was elected dean in 1943 and immediately went to work to achieve his goal: "a complete medical and health educational service and research center." In 1949, Dean Lynch's title was changed to president.

In 1952, the Medical College of the State of South Carolina enlarged its freshman medical class to eighty students and shortened its name to the Medical College of South Carolina. The College of Pharmacy moved to the fourth floor of the newly constructed Laboratory-Clinic Building (Cancer Clinic) and would soon occupy the entire building. By 1955, the new five-hundred-bed Medical College Hospital was completed. The new School of Nursing building followed the next year. At last, the Medical College achieved Class-A status. It would soon have a School of Dental Medicine (1967) and a School of Allied Health Professions (1968), and in 1969 it became the Medical University of South Carolina. But growth and change included turmoil and conflict.

POSTWAR STUDENT BOOM

As always, students were strapped for money. And in the prosperous 1950s, they had little trouble finding part-time work to help out. Dr. Charles H. Banov (class of 1955) recalled his unusual job in his memoir, *Office Upstairs: A Doctor's Journey*:

> As medical students, Julian [Atkinson] and I shared a special part-time job. On Saturday mornings, we were paid ten dollars to drive more than five hours to Columbia, the state capital, in the Medical College truck and bring back the cadavers of unclaimed bodies from the state mental hospital. In those days, there was no interstate highway, and we had to pick up some

ice to keep the cadavers cool. I'll always remember the look on the faces of the ice workers when we drove our truck in, opened the box and said, "Please give us a load of ice before we go fishing."

Dr. William Harvey Hunter (class of 1952) worked several jobs, some highly educational and some highly unusual, to support his wife and two children. He later described his work in an article in *The Journal of the South Carolina Medical Association*:

I made $100 a month riding the ambulance for Roper Hospital...We were 24 hours on duty and 24 hours off—this for the entire year. I probably was exposed to as much medicine riding this ambulance as in any other rotation in my medical education.

...Dr. H.R. Pratt-Thomas had a grant to try to determine the cause of cancer of the cervix. His thought was that Jewish women didn't have a lot of such cancers; that perhaps the smegma found within the foreskin of uncircumcised males may contribute to cancer of the cervix...To study this, Dr. Pratt-Thomas acquired 400 virgin cancer strain E white mice. He developed a vaginal speculum which included an insert that would smear smegma on the cervices of the mice...I literally did thousands of pelvic exams on virgin mice to work my way through medical school.

I had only one problem with this, which was to get enough smegma. Haunting the clinics at the medical school and the wards at old Roper with tongue blades, I scraped much smegma from any man who had a foreskin. Once when we ran short, we went up to the state asylum in Columbia where they lined up all the uncircumcised males, and I sat there with my tongue blades scraping away.

Postwar nursing students seemed more determined now to stretch the very tight boundaries placed on their activities. This continually raised the ire of Director of Nursing (later dean) Ruth Chamberlin, who wrote to the president of the Student Government Association in 1949:

To date the students are granted many privileges, but have not accepted their part of the bargain seriously concerning life in the home.
1.   Students are not in their own rooms and quiet at 10:30 pm.
2.   Students are continuously late and noisy in returning on 11 o'clock leaves.
3.   Radios are played after 10 pm.

4. Night nurses are not quiet when they come off duty.
5. Students are entertaining their friends in cars in front of the nurses home after 10 pm, thus disturbing occupants of Annex B, the Main Home and Riverside, whereas students have been repeatedly reminded that entertaining is not to be done in cars.

Some students of the postwar era resorted to the power of the pen to challenge the system. Under the pseudonym Titre J. Beakerdam, one College of Pharmacy poet protested his classes in general and Dr. J. Hampton Hoch in particular:

Do the teachers really think,
We don't know their techniques stink?
Better lectures have I heard,
From a coach way down on third.
'Taint enough we have to listen,
He calls the roll—we can't be missin'.

Go before "J.H. Contagion,"
Kills your youth's imagination.
Such contagion warps the soul,
Makes one sneaky like the mole.
Let me count the times I've wondered,
If J. Hampton ever blundered.
"Never!" says that pseudo-prince,
"Words like error make me wince."

As postwar students graduated, their lives beyond campus quickly introduced them to more serious responsibilities. Dr. Robert Phillips, for example, completed his residency at the Medical College in July 1957 and soon began work at a Presbyterian mission hospital in Korea. He wrote to Dr. Henry Frierson in 1958 about his experiences:

The country is still badly torn up from the war and there is scarcely a mile of pavement to be found outside Seoul and the big military establishments... The people are smart, contrary to reports from the GI's, and they have a terrific sense of humor. Some of the Korean house staff are astoundingly well grounded in the basic sciences and I would stack two or three of them up against any intern or resident I've seen in the States; all the surgical residents are quite good technicians. The Koreans are all good with their hands.

...Our pathology technician, a Korean triple amputee, makes quite good slides, but I am the pathologist and I wish I had learned more pathology. I also do the GI fluoroscopy and the endoscopy...My first radical neck patient died of a stroke on the third day. I had done a tongue-jaw-neck on him and he looked like a rose until the calamity. I've done one total gastrectomy, some ordinary stomachs, gall bladders, spleens, and one esophagus, some abdominal perineals, only one radical mastectomy, and lots of bone cases. Also I'm doing the obstetrics on the missionaries, and all has gone well so far...At last I've found a place where I can make rounds when I want to.

New Faces Arrive...Slowly

Although schools and hospitals were rigidly segregated, and women were mostly expected to be nurses or nursing faculty, diversity of gender, ethnicity and region (although not yet of race) made small inroads. Dr. Charles Banov recalled the uphill battle:

In 1951, my last year at Emory, the finish line was in sight. It wasn't hard to handicap the medical school horse race: few girls were ever accepted, blacks never were and at the Medical College of South Carolina, there was an unwritten but obvious rule that limited the number of Jewish applicants accepted. For the past hundred years there were usually two, but occasionally four, Jews accepted in any class. Every bright, Jewish, pre-med student in the state competed for those few places.

Dr. H. Biemann Othersen Jr. (class of 1953) recalled the single female student in his Medical School class of about sixty students:

She was very smart, number one in the class, drove a baby blue Cadillac convertible, and beat everyone at tennis. But she married her lab partner and dropped out of school.

Eventually, in the wake of the Supreme Court decision in *Brown v. Board of Education* (1954) and various state court rulings, some students and faculty began to question racial inequities. Dr. Layton McCurdy (class of 1960 and later chair of the department of psychiatry and dean of the College of Medicine) recalled his experiences in a speech to medical students in January 2008:

My awakening came in this hospital on 7-East. And by the way, the East floors were black and West floors were white. My awakening came, thanks to a charge nurse named Green...

After a particularly grueling evening of scut work, when the residents and interns had left for other adventures, I suggested to Mrs. Green that we go downstairs and partake in the free late night snack. She looked at me and said, "You and I don't eat in the same dining room." Mrs. Green was about my color which in many ways made my lesson more powerful. I didn't sleep much that night. I found myself reviewing the good times with my black friends, both my age and older and my willingness to buy into the argument that I had heard so many times, "We treat our black people well." Ironically, that was 1958 when Martin Luther King was emerging as a powerful spokesperson.

Faculty diversity at the School of Medicine began when Dr. Elsie Tabor was appointed assistant professor of anatomy, the first full-time female faculty member in that school. Promoted to professor in 1965 and teaching until 1980, she upheld the tradition of colorful anatomists, as Dr. Russell Harley recalled in an article in *Catalyst* (2000):

> Generations of medical students spent countless hours studying embryology under her tutelage, and I'll bet there are still a lot of fetal pig drawings out there somewhere. Her articulation was reminiscent of Katherine Hepburn... and she would sometimes open her mouth to speak and then just hold it there while everybody waited to find out what she was going to say. She was quite approachable, but still, she was always the teacher in control.

Dr. Tabor introduced human genetics to the embryology course for first-year medical students and was widely credited with improving the quality of education at the Medical College. In 1974, she was instrumental in reforming the curriculum. At one meeting she announced:

> I was given the dubious honor of addressing you tonight to describe our present curriculum. This seemed necessary because there are many newcomers on our faculty...who don't know what it is all about. Also there is an even larger group of old timers who still don't know what the hell it's all about.

Once very scarce, another face increasing in number during the postwar years was the faculty member from "off." Dr. William H. Golod, appointed to the Pharmacy faculty in 1958 and later dean of the College of Pharmacy, recalled his serendipitous move, after receiving his PhD at Purdue University, as an experience with a gracious southern welcome:

> When I interviewed at campuses in the spring, I told them I wanted no classes Friday afternoons and Monday mornings, because I was still running marathons for the New York Athletic Club and wanted to be able to travel to them and back when necessary on weekends. That wasn't such a welcome idea at most places; they'd just look at me and snarl, "You can't decide when you won't be available to teach classes." But here at the Medical College, Dean [William Allen] Prout was just a kindly Kentucky gentleman who said, "Oh, that's just fine. Just wonderful. Looks like you are coming here with a grant that will come with you and with good training. Ah, that's just fine." So I came here, trained on the streets and at the Citadel track and kept running those weekend marathons.

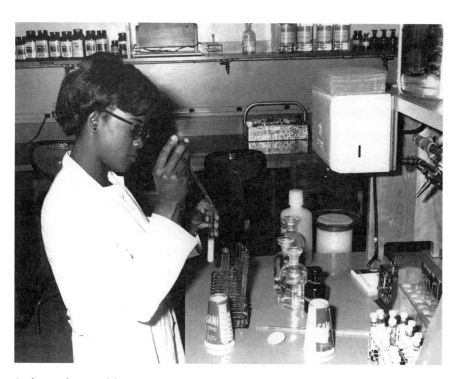

Student in chemistry laboratory. *Waring Historical Library, MUSC.*

Dr. Othersen experienced a reverse sense of being from "off" when he moved North after graduating from the Medical School:

> When I graduated, I drove around the country interviewing for an internship. There was a tradition that the first and second honor grads went to Cincinnati. The doctor who interviewed me there said, "So you're from South Carolina? Amazing what you turn out with what you have." I went to Philadelphia General where there were about 109 interns, and we found we could compete with them...I came back to MUSC [in 1965] because all Charlestonians come back. I was the first pediatric surgeon in South Carolina when I came on the faculty...My first patient was a distant cousin who wanted her ears pierced. I charged her two dollars, and I wanted to frame those first bills; but I needed the two dollars.

Palliatives for Financial Needs

As a dean and then a president, Dr. Lynch was persistent and innovative in developing funding sources for the Medical College. Dean Golod recalled:

> Dr. Lynch was a very unique person. In the 1940's, he was the only board certified pathologist in the state. So, he convinced the hospital accreditors that they should insist that pathological specimens taken in every hospital in the state should be examined by a board certified pathologist. They agreed, and since the hospitals didn't have their own pathologists, all specimens were coming to the Medical College Pathology Department constantly. The money that came in with them was significant. This went on for about a dozen years and was a key to the survival of the Medical College at the time.

The era of research grants and contracts was beginning, but some at the Medical College worried about the consequences of soft funding. Dr. Golod brought with him a five-year grant from the National Institutes of Health, as well as contracts with pharmaceutical firms. But he found mixed reactions:

> It was really a sleepy medical college campus. And after a year of that grant here, Dr. Lynch told me: "We don't take Yankee dollars here." He insisted that I give the rest of the grant back. At that point, research just wasn't so attractive to administrators, because they couldn't really control

it or the people doing it. They also were wary of the strings that might be attached by funders.

Yet change happened quickly, and by 1966, when William McCord was named president, outside funding was an essential component of vital research. Dr. Peter C. Gazes (class of 1944), the first board-certified cardiologist in South Carolina, had joined the Medical College faculty in 1950. He later recalled:

> We were underfunded, but we got on the map with President McCord. Dr. McCord, he was something else. We called him Whip. He would take me to Columbia and have me sit in the front row at the meetings of the Ways and Means Committee—because many of them were my patients. Then he would party with them at the old Wade Hampton Hotel. He turned the tide.

And Then the Revolution

The year 1968 was by any reckoning extraordinary: the assassinations of Dr. Martin Luther King Jr. and Robert F. Kennedy, urban riots, protest rallies on college campuses. At the Medical College, 1968 didn't happen until 1969. Then, workers' rights and civil rights coincided in a mix that proved explosive.

The "nonprofessional" hospital workers at the Medical College Hospital wanted to organize with hospital union 1199B, which had been in town for a year trying to unionize workers at several hospitals. President McCord had made his position on unions clear in a memo to employees the previous year:

> October 14, 1968
> Dear Fellow Employees:
> ...In order that there be no misunderstanding as to exactly where the Medical College stands on this union matter, I want to make our position crystal clear. WE DO NOT WANT A UNION HERE AT THE MEDICAL COLLEGE. It is our sincere belief that this union [Local 15a Retail, Wholesale, and Tobacco Workers Union] has nothing worthwhile or constructive to offer any of you.
> This union is interested in one thing and one thing only. That's MONEY. YOUR MONEY!...We of course, consider this union matter to be extremely serious. It will affect both you and your family. It could affect you and your job here at the Medical College.

FOR THIS REASON IT IS OUR INTENTION TO RESIST THIS UNION IN ITS ATTEMPT TO GET IN HERE WITH EVERY LEGAL MEANS AT OUR DISPOSAL—MAKE NO MISTAKE ABOUT THAT.
Yours very sincerely,
William M. McCord, M.D., Ph.D.
President

The workers hoping to unionize were led by nurses' aide Mary Moultrie, whose professional situation, taken later in a formal complaint statement, seemed all too familiar to other nonprofessional workers:

I, Miss Mary Moultrie, worked as a nurses' aide at the Medical College Hospital. I was employed on the date of March 10, 1966 to March 17, 1969. Starting salary for me was seventy cents per hour which over a period of approximately two years, six months, became $1.33 per hour. No definite reason was given for my not receiving higher wages, although I questioned it many times, I brought it to the attention of the vice president of the hospital and other administrators including the assistant director of nursing...There was a white nurses' aide, employed 2½ years later than I had been and was making more money. She started with Nurses' Aide Technician pay which at that time was $1.54 per hour. I was only making $1.33 per hour.

Pressured by Charleston mayor R. Palmer Galliard, Dr. McCord invited a small group of disgruntled workers to meet with him; but he was soon confronted with eighty unhappy employees and refused to meet with such a large group. Twelve of the group were summarily fired, including Mary Moultrie, who explained:

I was invited to attend a meeting March 17, 1969 with the president of Medical College Hospital, Dr. W.M. McCord, which resulted in my dismissal. On March 17, at 10 o'clock I left my unit with permission...I returned to the floor at 12 o'clock and resumed my work. At 3:20 the seventh floor supervisor Mrs. Burney came to me and asked me to report to Nursing service at 3:30 p.m. which was at the end of the work day. I arrived at 3:30 and was confronted by the Director of Nursing, Mrs. Jo Ann Lowder and the Seventh Floor Supervisor, Mrs. Louise Burney. There I was told that I had left critically ill patients unattended for more than an hour and was therefore terminated.
Mary Ann Moultrie
National Organizing Committee

The strike was on! Dr. Layton McCurdy remembered:

> Many hospital workers walked out. The hospital staff went down to skeleton force. The job was to keep the hospital open. Threats of violence started against people in the black community who continued to come to work. There were pickets and soon the National Guard was here with a curfew. Special passes were required to come into the hospital after curfew hours. You couldn't be on the streets. A few of our students joined the picket lines.

Newspaper headlines told the story:

Charleston Evening Post, March 28, 1969
"County Hospital Workers Picket"

Charleston News and Courier, April 1, 1969
"Abernathy Pledges Support to Strikers"

Charleston News and Courier, April 2, 1969
"McNair Says State Can't Bargain"

Charleston News and Courier, April 3, 1969
"McCord Rejects Clergy Committee's Peace Proposal"

Charleston News and Courier, April 5, 1969
"Peaceful March Staged by Strikers"

New York Times, April 21, 1969
"14 Rights Leaders Support Strikers"

Charleston News and Courier, April 22, 1969
"Abernathy Sets Mass March Against Struck Hospitals"

Charleston News and Courier, April 26, 1969
"Guardsmen Ordered into Tense Charleston"

Charleston News and Courier, April 28, 1969
"47 Are Arrested in Hospital March"

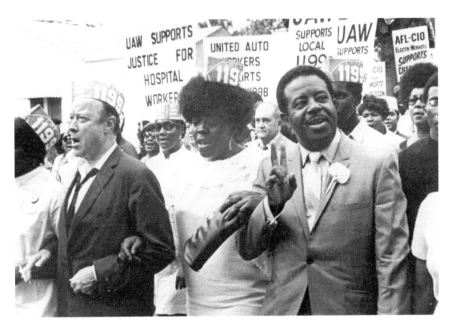

Above: Walter Reuther, Mary Moultrie and Ralph Abernathy in the hospital workers' strike, 1969. *Courtesy of Avery Research Center.*

Below, from left: Mrs. Leon Davis, Mary Moultrie, Coretta Scott King and three unidentified women in the march. *Courtesy of Avery Research Center.*

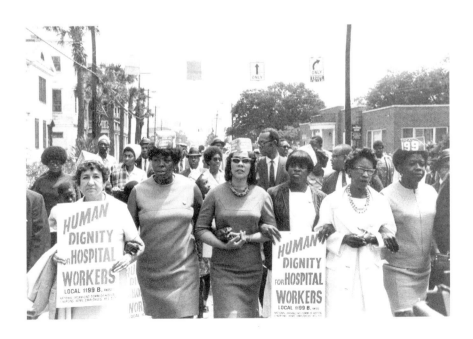

New York Times, April 29, 1969
"Charleston Is Armed Camp as 142 More Are Held"

Charleston News and Courier, May 1, 1969
"Widow of Dr. King Leads 1,500 on Hospital March"

Charleston News and Courier, May 2, 1969
"Curfew Imposed to 'Cool Down' Tense Charleston"

New York Times, May 3, 1969
"Abernathy Asks Nixon for Help in Hospital Strike"

Charleston News and Courier, May 10, 1969
"Nixon to Send Observers to Strike Scene"

New York Times, May 12, 1969
"12,000 March in Charleston in Support of Hospital Strikers"

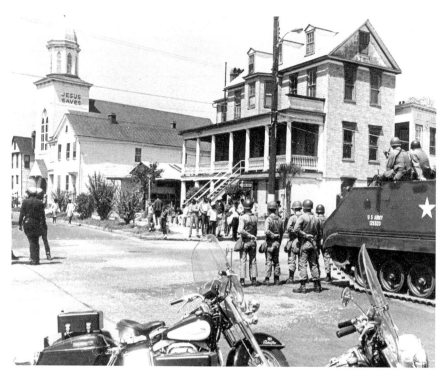

The National Guard in Charleston during the hospital strike. *Courtesy of Avery Research Center.*

Charleston News and Courier, June 28, 1969
"Medical College Strike Ends after 100 Days"

In a terse announcement, President McCord confirmed the end of the strike:

> All those working on March 17 will return to their jobs on Tuesday. A grievance procedure has been set up and they can have a credit union.

THE MEANING OF A UNIVERSITY

Ironically, a proposal to change the name of the Medical College went forward to the legislature during the strike, and on July 1, the Medical College of South Carolina became the Medical University of South Carolina. The former schools within it became colleges.

The strike wasn't the first sign of civil rights consciousness in Charleston. Racial diversity came to campus as a number of pioneering students arrived. Charleston native Bernard Deas, who became the first African American graduate of the Medical College in 1971, entered in 1966 after graduating from Iowa State University as an ROTC Distinguished Military Graduate. Dr. Deas later recalled:

> It was very interesting how my going to MUSC unfolded. At Iowa State, I majored in bacteriology and intended to work in a lab as a medical researcher. By about junior year, I got tired of just being in a lab with a microscope. I wanted to be with people. Some things came together then. For one thing, I was sick and missed a quarter. My physician, a wonderful young black doctor back in Charleston, was killed in an auto accident at that time. He had been such a light for that profession and its diversity to come. Then, I found out my father always wanted to be a physician. He was a letter carrier, and he'd put me and my two sisters through college. He really sacrificed. My mother explained to me how much he would be proud to have me become a doctor; he had always wanted that for himself, but his parents couldn't afford to send him to college. With much reflection, I started thinking about becoming a physician.
>
> The year before I enrolled, there were one or two black females who enrolled but didn't come back for sophomore year. I don't know why. So, when I came along as the next black student, I sort of half expected there to

be a big deal about my enrollment. But the Medical University just accepted me. There may have been some people who didn't want me there, but if there were, they kept their mouths shut.

Also, even though my home was in Charleston, I decided it was best for me to live in the dormitory. I made friends. We went to class together, shot pool together, ate in the cafeteria together. We'd go to pitch and putt golf together, which was a good way to take out frustrations.

The hospital strike took on extra meaning for Dr. Deas:

I was very worried when the hospital workers started picketing. I thought that going to class, I'd look like someone who was a potential picketer crossing the picket line—even though I was wearing my white coat and tie. I remember walking between picketing people saying, "I'm a student here. Excuse me, I have to go to class."

Forty years later, Dr. Deas recalled teachers and mentors:

Dr. Elsie Tabor gave lectures that were always captivating. She came across as a tough person, but soon there was always some levity involved in her classrooms. She had a sense of humor. She seemed to have something she needed to prove—to show she could run with the big dogs. But we also realized that she had a lighter side.

Dr. Pratt-Thomas was so smart. You just sat there in awe of his knowledge and his teaching ability.

The most interesting was Dr. Metcalf, an anatomy instructor. He had been a professor at the Citadel. He adopted me and a student named Ben Simmons, and he'd take us out for lunch breaks. We'd go to the Citadel pool. He really imparted social wisdom to us—about life, focusing, persevering. He was soft spoken and introspective—willing to share. But, back on campus he was our anatomy professor; we still had to pass the exams like everyone else.

So I had contacts and mentors. And when I felt I needed to be reminded of my roots, I got on my bicycle and rode the six blocks home.

(After completing his internship, residency and fellow appointments with the regular army commission he had earned as an undergraduate, Dr. Deas served in the army as both a physician and a medical administrator in Texas, Georgia and New Mexico. He retired in 1994.)

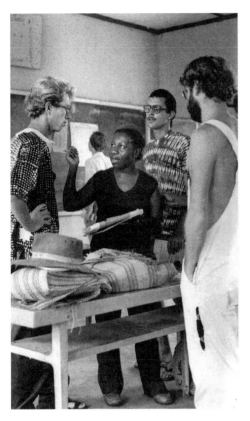

Dr. Delores Gibbs (class of 1973) training new Peace Corps volunteers in Sierra Leone, where she served as the sole Peace Corps physician. *Courtesy of Delores Gibbs.*

Dr. Rose Delores Gibbs (class of 1973) also modeled the way for diverse students. A graduate of Fisk University and a South Carolina native, she began a lifelong dream of becoming a doctor when she entered the Medical College in 1968 with 124 fellow students. Among the 7 women, only 1 was African American—Rose Delores Gibbs. She later reflected on her experiences:

> When I left high school, I thought I was smart. Then I got to Fisk, and my fellow students seemed so smart. Then I got to MUSC, and everyone seemed super smart! I was competing with a lot of brain matter. So, I had to study hard, but I enjoyed that. I made some friends, although I didn't really do a lot of socializing. John Cross, who moved from Pharmacy to Medicine, and his wife Ann were my closest friends. We'd go to lunch and dinner and movies together. On Saturdays, I'd often come home to Moncks Corner.

Being a pioneering student could include difficulties outside of class. Dr. Gibbs recalled:

> I wanted to live close to campus, but I had problems finding a place to rent in the area. I went to one perfect and available house; when I showed up, I was told it was already rented. A friend of mine called about it later and was told it was still for rent. He was really overcome on my behalf and wanted us to take legal action, or at least go to the housing authority. I thought and really just decided: Hold off. I'm not here in Charleston to solve the housing

problem for all of us. I'm here to be in medical school, so let's just leave it be. I ended up living West of the Ashley; I didn't want to live there, but I had to.

Supportive faculty were key:

Dr. Arthur Williams, a nephrologist, helped me when I was having trouble discerning figures and details on slides of the microscope. He told me that since I could sew and embroider, I had an advantage over the male students; I was used to working with very small figures. He advised me to think about embroidery when I looked through the microscope, searching for tiny patterns. It worked! Dr. Elsie Tabor was tough and very smart. I respected her. Dr. Kathleen Riley, a dermatologist, would take the girls for beach cookouts, and she had no problem including me.

I did have one memorable experience on an obstetrics rotation. Each of us was assigned to a woman in labor—to follow her progress and assist with the delivery. The chief resident, making rounds with four of my classmates, came in while I was doing an examination. And he started chewing me out—in a way that I could tell he thought I was a nurses' aide. I had to tell him I was a medical student. He didn't apologize...A few weeks later, he came in while I was in the gynecology clinic; and he spent about 30 minutes with me, showing me things, really teaching me. I think it was his way of saying he was sorry.

After graduation and completing an internal medicine residency, Gibbs went to Sierra Leone with the Peace Corps, and her education continued:

I was the only Peace Corps physician there. I was surprised how well trained African doctors and nurses were—they had trained in the U.S., England, Russia or China. But the problem was what you had to work with: Limited supplies, medications, immunizations, respirators and such. No advanced life care units. I quickly realized that health education and preventive medicine were the tools doctors needed. Because there is so little corrective surgery and prevention, you see everything. You get to see all the complications of T.B., leprosy, rabies, polio, river blindness, tetanus. You see all the stages of a disease process that you will never see back here; it is terrible, but extraordinary.

(Dr. Gibbs later traveled around the world as chief of medical operations for the Peace Corps. Eventually, she returned to Berkeley County, South Carolina, where she opened her own medical practice.)

James Hodges entered the Pharmacy School in 1967 as its first African American student. Now the owner and pharmacist at Cash Discount Drug Store in St. George, South Carolina, he recalled in an interview that being a "first" was less important than conquering rigorous academics:

> When I became an undergraduate at Claflin College, I started looking around. One day, Dean Golod was a speaker at the college, and he told us about pharmacy education at MUSC, and I thought, "This is what I'm going to do." Dean Golod went through the prerequisites, the courses you had to have taken, and I went back and looked at my courses. I'd taken all of them!
>
> I was going to a school for a reason, and that was to become a pharmacist. Who was and wasn't there, that was a society issue...I had the desire, but I had to get into a mindset of how the math worked, how this and that should and shouldn't be done. Probably about thirty pharmacy students started, and about fifteen graduated. I think we had about five women. I liked the rigor. It really made me appreciate the profession. There was a precision—never an "almost." There was fairness and no exceptions.

Some students returned to school after professional experience, entering MUSC because they could. Among them was Rosslee Green Douglas, who had attended Dillard University and Lincoln School of Nursing and had worked in home healthcare nursing in New York and South Carolina. In 1972, she became the first African American graduate of the College of Nursing (BS). She later explained her practical motivations:

> When I went to Dillard, the nursing schools were segregated. Most of the people who were considered minorities were nurses' aides. Eventually, if you were white, you could get a B.S.N.; and you were in charge. I had a lot of experiences with visiting nurse services in New York and home health services in South Carolina. I heard the girls at MUSC were now graduating with Bachelor degrees, and I decided I needed a little something extra.
>
> I was surrounded by much younger students, and I had credits from Dillard and Lincoln and NYU. So I really wasn't at MUSC very long. I didn't see other students of color, although there might have been some just starting. It [the BS degree] helped a whole lot. It made me more credible in a sense. As a black individual, you had to establish yourself...I decided that extra was what I had to do.

(In 1981, Rosslee Douglas became the first African American female appointee of the Reagan administration when Secretary of Energy James Edwards selected her to head his department's Office of Minority Economic Impact. She received an honorary doctor of humane letters degree from MUSC in 1985.)

Another pioneering group of students was the first class enrolled in the School of Dental Medicine in 1967, with twenty-one receiving DMD degrees in 1971. Their first dean, Dr. John E. Buhler, arrived in 1964 from Emory University and then private industry to lay the foundation. He wrote a former colleague:

> October 28, 1965
> Dear Bill:
> ...I'm getting along here splendidly—we have a big house—et cetera—and all of that. But I'll be honest and tell you I have not by any means found my return to education as gratifying as I thought it would be. Actually, Bill, in addition to being Dean of the Dental School, I am also the Coordinator of Planning and Development for the entire Medical College, including Schools of Medicine, Pharmacy, Nursing, Graduate Studies and the Medical College Hospital...I tell you this because I want you to know that things here are going splendidly.

D. Edward (Eddie) Collins Jr., a freshman dental student in 1970 and later a faculty member, recalled the circumstances of those early Dental College years:

> The College of Dental Medicine was housed in historic Colcock Hall, a building newly renovated and serving now as administrative offices for the entire university. The Dental College/Basic Science Building was under construction at that time. Colcock Hall was not air conditioned back then and the cramped laboratories were sweltering—especially when we had four dozen Bunsen burners going.
> In the first two years of school we had to shape and place practice "fillings" in plastic teeth. The student who sat next to me in lab would always do a little carving, then blow on the tooth to clean off debris. The first time he treated a real patient, he did the same thing in the patient's mouth—much to her dismay!
> Cathy Moss was the only female in our class and the first female to be admitted. She hung in there like the rest of us and we loved her like a sister.

Some dental students from out of state were noticeable for their Yankee accents, so the Dental College newsletter, *The Mouthpiece*, published a "Column of Charlestonese (for those from off)" in 1972, including these definitions:

"Ice cool"—The institution of learning which stands midway between grammar school and college.
"Lack"—Enjoy, i.e., "I lack fried chicken."
"Lawn"—Not short.
"Bare"—A beverage from malt and hops.
"Poet"—To transfer a liquid, i.e., "Poet from the pitcher to the glass."
"Layman"—A fruit from which layman-ade is made.
"Ain't"—Sister of one of your parents.
"Balks"—A container, such as a match balks.
"Luck"—To direct one's gaze, i.e., "Luck year, Pappa, what Bubber done to your match balks."
"Poke"—Hog meat.

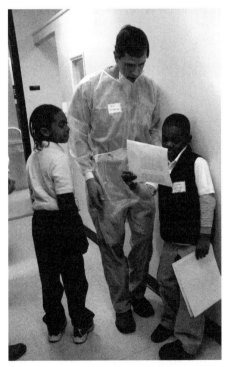

Give Kids a Smile Day. Dental student Ben Massey shows Jordan Washington, seven, a copy of his X-ray. *Courtesy of Office of Public Relations, MUSC.*

Student voices were sounding in university communities everywhere. At MUSC, even the once constrained nursing students began to speak their minds. In their 1973 student newsletter, *The Prognosis*, Linda Smith and Joan Moore wrote a letter, "To Whom It May Concern":

We are expressing our concern over the unfair treatment of our students in the nursing department. This past week approx. 7 students were told to either write a paper using modified footnotes and 5 references OR to have 5 points taken off of our final grade. This was done because these students left a class early and missed a lecture. Before leaving, the students told the instructors

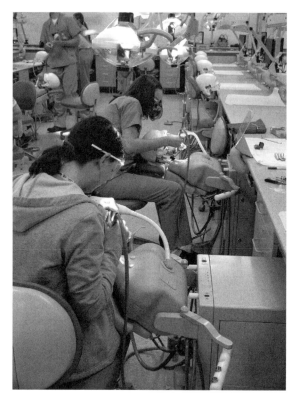

Left: Dental students with mannequins. *Courtesy of College of Dental Medicine, MUSC.*

Below: College of Charleston biology class prepares aspiring medical students. *Courtesy of Special Collections, College of Charleston Libraries.*

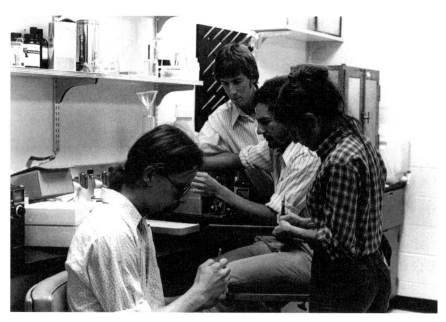

they needed to leave and the instructor replied, "Use your own discretion."...
We feel this "assignment" was given for punitive reasons, but the instructor
stated that this assignment is the only way to make up what we missed, and
that it was for our own good...If this is a university in 1973, I fail to see it...

We are taught to think for ourselves, but if our thoughts or views go
against the grain then they are wrong...I respect you if you do not agree,
though. I realize this will do no good for the 7 "examples," but I hope it will
move a few people to think about how we are all being treated. "YOU DO
HAVE RIGHTS."

CHAPTER 8

SIMULATION, CYBERSPACE
AND SPECIALIZATION

The decade after the tumultuous strike began with promise. Dr. James W. Colbert had joined the faculty as the first vice-president and provost, and he envisioned a new integration of medical education and medical research to make MUSC a nationally recognized academic institution. He began by recruiting prominent researchers. One of the first was his friend Dr. Albert Sabin, famous for developing the live polio vaccine that eliminated the crippling disease in America.

SUPERSTAR PROFESSOR

Dr. Sabin, the first distinguished research professor of biomedicine, talked about teaching at MUSC—when he was in town—in a 1977 interview:

> I give lectures to students here...I enjoy it because I love to look into the faces of students and imagine myself almost 50 years back...I want to transmit to them not only facts which they must have for their professional training. I want to transmit to them also the excitement of how facts are obtained...I will put down on a page or two pages the things they should remember, but I want them to *listen to me*. We have a very gratifying experience together, and that is what I enjoy. I give quite a number of lectures here during the year, although perhaps not as many as I give in other schools around the country and abroad.

Dr. H. Biemann Othersen Jr. (class of 1953), professor of pediatric surgery, remembered the importance of Dr. Sabin's arrival:

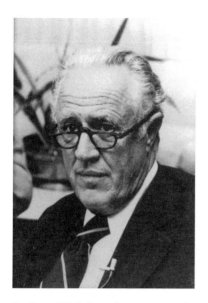

Dr. James W. Colbert, first provost and vice-president of academic affairs, 1969. *Courtesy of Office of Public Relations, MUSC.*

There's a good story about Sabin who was a courtly looking gentleman and came down here as a distinguished professor. The idea was to use his impetus to build research further. One day a doctor in Walhalla called the president and told him that a Dr. John W. Wickliffe from West Union had invested in Georgia Pacific and had left all his money to his unmarried daughter Margaret who was looking around for philanthropy. So the president went up to talk to her and took Sabin along because he was such a great man. When Miss Wickliffe saw him she said, "Why he looks just like Daddy!" and sat down and wrote the check that bought Wickliffe House.

Dr. Colbert, however, had little time to realize his vision; he was killed in a plane crash in 1974. Charlene Stuart, former vice-president for finance and administration and Medical Center CFO, remembered:

On September 11, 1974, MUSC had its personal "9/11"! I remember feeling immense sorrow and grief while at the same time I was unable to comprehend the loss of such a great leader and his two sons. The entire administrative staff was stunned, and little did we know how difficult the next ten years would be for MUSC. Dr. Colbert laid groundwork for the success of MUSC today. More importantly, he inspired all with whom he worked to think bigger than South Carolina. He touched my career and the careers of my mentors with his belief in national excellence...We had never dared to dream about what he convinced us we could achieve.

A President with a Problem

Dr. William H. Knisely (class of 1954) was named president in 1975 and progress stopped. Dr. Othersen recalled the bad press that ensued:

Dr. William Knisely and his older brother Dr. Melvin Knisely, the anatomy professor, came together—we called them the Chicago mob. They set up a lab with graduate students, another step towards being a research institution. But in the late 1970's when Knisely was president, the press just went after MUSC. He just couldn't deal with them. They jumped on us for everything. Channel 5 was even being paid a retainer but they were particularly vicious. In 1982, Jim Edwards was named president and he fed on the press, a born politician.

A President with a History

Dr. James Burrows Edwards had already served as governor of South Carolina (1975–79) and a Reagan cabinet member (U.S. secretary of energy, 1981–82) when he accepted the presidency of the Medical University. An oral surgeon and World War II veteran, Dr. Edwards quickly demonstrated the advantages of bringing high-level experience and multifaceted talents to the office as he set about fundraising for two of his priorities: endowing faculty chairs and improving physical facilities:

> When I came here in 1982, there were one and a half endowed chairs. I realized that with a chair, I could attract outstanding clinicians from all over the world. It's a wonderful way to get great faculty—dangle an endowed chair and the Charleston lifestyle...When I left, there were 28 chairs fully funded. Now, there are about 40.

The hospital caught Edwards's attention early, and he launched a vigorous campaign to fund improvements:

> I went to the ward on the tenth floor, where the psychiatric patients were located. It hadn't been painted in so long, and the furniture was all torn up and ragged. I said, "We're going to close this." Then I got the Institute of Psychiatry.
>
> When General Mark Clark was here in his final illness, his wife was greeting visitors from around the world in this awful hallway. The real opinion makers in the state didn't want to come to the Medical University. I decided we could build a private pavilion, if not with state funding, then with private funding. We wanted four little apartments on the four corners of the hospital, each with a room for the patient and a room for the family. In

about two nights of calling, we raised $7 million for the Palmetto Pavilion. With people donating for specific rooms, at one point I mentioned to Ann, "I'm in trouble. I've sold five corners of a four sided building!" The Palmetto Pavilion uplifted the whole state of mind of clinical faculty, and it influenced the other floors too.

And then the southern touch:

I realized we needed to do better in the people area, so I said we all have to take a course in hospitality. The doctors thought it was sophomoric, but they did it. Actually, I had to hire a company from Pittsburgh to teach southern hospitality!

Dr. Edwards's summation:

I loved every minute at MUSC. There were so many things to get done. Building, creating, making progress—when you get into a mode like that, it's uplifting. I just loved it.

During Dr. Edwards's seventeen-year presidency, the campus area increased three-fold, the budget increased six-fold and research funding increased from an estimated $5 million to $90 million.

MUSC Gets Teeth...Some Real, Some Plastic

The new College of Dental Medicine established itself as the right school for South Carolina dentists. Dr. Edward "Eddie" Collins joined the faculty in 1974 as an instructor of operative dentistry. His students were particularly memorable for their work in labs, technical and simulated:

There was a student of mine who was prone not to keep her wits about her. In technique lab she caught her hair on fire twice in two weeks with the Bunsen burner. It filled the lab with a horrible odor. That same semester, she got her hair caught in the long belt that drove the handpiece ("drill") and we had to reverse it to unravel her hair. She graduated anyway.

In the simulation lab, students have been known to screw up. Like they do the wrong tooth, but better they do it in the lab than on live patients. We

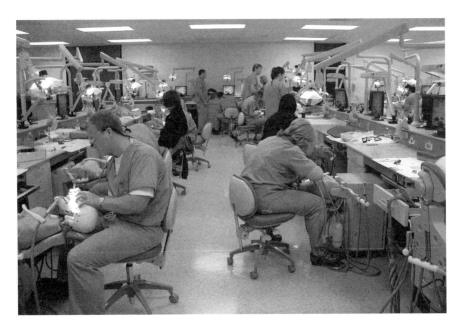

Dental students with mannequins. *Courtesy of College of Dental Medicine, MUSC.*

use simulated heads with simulated teeth in them with simulated cavities under color-corrected lighting.

Students transitioned from plastic teeth to real ones:

In my introduction to dentistry course for freshman, I refer to myself as a coach. The first two years of dental school are basic science and technique (on plastic teeth) courses. The last two are in the patient care clinic. Students also work in free clinics like the East Cooper Community Outreach and many go on missionary trips.

What makes a good day is to see the light go on when a student finally grasps something that is challenging. I was smiling widely the first year our entering freshmen had a higher GPA than the College of Medicine's first year students. A lot of our students come from little tiny towns and go back to little tiny towns. And I have taught many children of students; I plan to retire when I come to their grandchildren.

Dr. Elizabeth Pilcher (class of 1981) remembered her days as a female dental student:

I was in the first four-year class. We were seven women out of 56 and very much a minority. So if one of us missed class, it was pretty obvious. The boys had to wear ties, but they weren't sure what we should wear. The Dean suggested nurses' uniforms but we talked him out of that!

I switched from pre med because I realized that dentistry was a good career for a woman. It made more sense to have a dentist's hours. I remember Dr. Hastings showed me the anatomy lab and said, "Don't be scared, honey."

Dr. Pilcher became a full-time faculty member in 1989 in the Department of Crown and Bridge (now the Department of Oral Rehabilitation):

I was the only woman faculty member for a long time. Now 25% of the faculty is female and 50% of the student body. And we have an association for women dentists.

Dr. Pilcher talked about recent changes in teaching:

When making a crown, we used to take an impression of the tooth, send it to the lab, get it back and put in the crown a couple of weeks later. Now it is possible for a camera to take an optical impression that goes straight to a computer which mills the tooth out of a block of tooth-colored porcelain, and it goes back in the same day.

This optical imaging will also change the way we teach. In the preclinical simulation lab we use a typodont—a plastic set of teeth that the students use to practice their preparations. Instructors look at each one and grade it visually. With the new technology, we will insert a camera on a wand, take an optical impression, and the computer will compare the work to a set of ideal measurements and grade it.

...The last ten or fifteen years have seen a new emphasis on cosmetic dentistry. People who used to wear dentures, now have implant supported dentures that are way more secure—a huge improvement. We have a very active implant division at the College now.

False teeth are gone and so is gold. Dr. Edward (Ted) Welsh, professor emeritus of restorative dentistry, noted its demise:

I was the last one to teach the use of gold. It is an art, like making full dentures. It's easy to do a gold crown, but an inlay or an onlay is difficult. It's labor intensive and requires real craftsmanship.

Charleston's Cardiologist

While nationally known medical researchers were joining the faculty at MUSC, some of their own were achieving national recognition. Dr. Peter C. Gazes (class of 1944), a faculty member since 1950, was establishing a reputation as a brilliant cardiologist as well as a caring and colorful teacher:

> One time I gave an exam and a student wrote for one of the answers, "Only God knows the answer to this question." So I wrote on his exam: God, 100. You, zero. Another time I gave students a long case about a patient who was traveling around, exhibiting many symptoms. I asked, "What would you do for this patient?" One student wrote: "Call Dr. Gazes in for consultation." I gave him 100.
>
> Tom Rowland [Dr. Thomas Clifford Rowland Jr., class of 1959], who later served as Chairman of the Board of Trustees, came to my office after his senior year and said, "I want to thank you for your teaching. And I want to have you as my cardiologist." I said, "By the time you have chest pain, you won't be able to afford me."

Dr. Gazes wrote his own textbook, *Clinical Cardiology: A Bedside Approach*, which went through four editions, and the Gazes Research Institute Building was named for him in 1996. He is renowned among medical students for what he can discern by inspection. He explained:

> I am one of the few bedside cardiologists left. I go into the room, examine the patient, take the history. The students must appreciate all the physical findings. Then we leave the room, and I say, "Now I will tell you what the echocardiogram will show." I'm trying to impress on them the importance of doing a good history and a good exam. Then they will know when to order an EKG and an echocardiogram—those are expensive. We can't do away with bedside care. I have patients who say their doctors don't listen to them. My motto is: Be scientific to the disease, but humane to the patient.

Decades of Doctors

Dr. Gazes reflected on medical students then and now:

> In the 1960's and 70's medical students were a bunch of mavericks. I mean they looked really, really bad; their appearance was unkempt. One I recall

had a beard that covered his whole face. I told him he looked like an armpit with teeth. He shaved it off. In my day we had to have a tie and a white coat and look decent. These students appeared in short sleeves, open shirts, hair exposed on their chests. It began changing in the 80s and 90's. Now they look like us again. They are perfectly groomed and very bright; they have been exposed to so much.

His colleague, Dr. Othersen, remembered his own medical school experience compared to the students of today:

When I was coming along, we students were all in the water hanging onto the sides of the pool, and the faculty would come along and step on our fingers. Then we would sink and bob up again; my first and second years were about surviving. In Dr. McCord's class in biochemistry the seating was alphabetical and I sat next to a Nelson who flunked out at mid-term. Thereafter I would look at that empty seat and break out in a sweat.

And our honor medical fraternity Alpha Omega Alpha met once a year for a banquet where we got drunk and told raunchy stories. Now the students have taken over the group, they meet every month and help

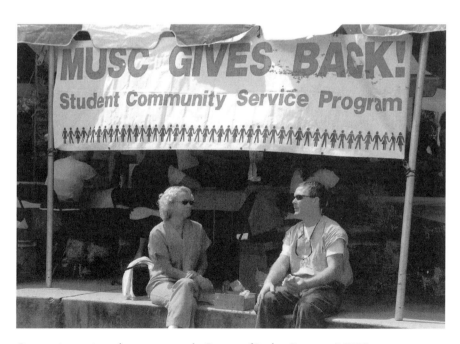

Community service and campus outreach. *Courtesy of Student Programs, MUSC.*

organize a variety of activities and events—the Charity Ball raised over $40,000 this year. The students are concerned with social issues. They run the CARES clinic over in East Cooper. And they have a real concern for medicine.

I want a clinician who can also do research. The foundation has to be good clinical care. You can solve the other problems. The patient has to be the most important voice at MUSC.

CHRONIC REALITIES OF PACE AND STRESS

What hasn't changed is the exhaustion that medical students experience. Dr. Anthony Colacino (class of 2009) felt like this one day:

I Want to Work in a Hospital

I want to work in a hospital
where there are wolves in the nursery
gobbling down the fresh-faced babes
as they take their questioning first breath
fur smeared with bright new blood

I want to work in a hospital
where the dead and near dying
are held hand-and-foot
and pitched from the roof
heavy sacks of flesh and bowels
trailing their lines as they plummet
and land in piles of broken marionettes

I want to work in a hospital
where the mentally challenged
follow trails of candy down sloping floors
to dim holes in the center of the room
Where a switch is flipped
chattering, glittering knives dance
and they are reduced to a howling porridge

Then he explained himself:

I'm a 36-year old in medicine as a second career after seven years of running an ice cream store/sub shop on Folly Beach, South Carolina. Long ago as an undergraduate at NYU, I had notions of writing. The prompt in our writing class was the line "I want to work in a hospital," the title of a poem by Cortney Davis. I opted for expressing the fatigue and disillusionment many of us feel as we end medical school, when empathy is dangerously low and we are sick of patients and the grind in general. I think everyone in medical school experiences these feelings at some point, but we keep them to ourselves.

The poem's tone was intended to be a cross between evoking a visceral response (shock value, if you will) and satire. I would be aghast if anyone actually took it seriously. It's just a way of expressing that there are days in medicine where you wish you could march a particularly demanding, obnoxious, arrogant, needy, self-destructive, abusive patient up to the roof and toss him off, and go home and have a cold beer and watch the waves roll in on the beach.

PROGNOSIS: SPECIALIZATION AND SPECIALIZED HELPERS

As twentieth- (now twenty-first-) century medicine became increasingly specialized, doctors needed increasingly specialized technical support. A new college developed to provide it. Catherine McCullough, director of development for the College of Health Professions, explained its history and mission:

The College began in 1966 as the College of Allied Health Professions, and it was scattered all over campus. Now we are all housed together in this wonderful building, the old High School of Charleston, saved from becoming a parking lot—much to the relief of its alums—and beautifully renovated. We saved the high school's motto too: "Enter to learn; leave to serve."

Our programs are always changing to meet current needs. The Department of Health Professions trains nurse anesthetists and cardiovascular perfusionsts, occupational and physical therapists, physicians assistants, and health administrators; and the Department of Health Sciences and Research offers graduate degrees in health leadership, research administration, and health and rehabilitation science. You might say that

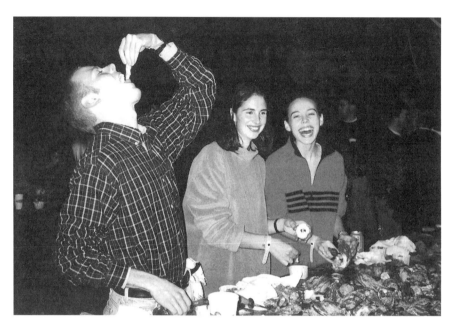

Students enjoy an oyster roast. *Courtesy of Student Programs, MUSC.*

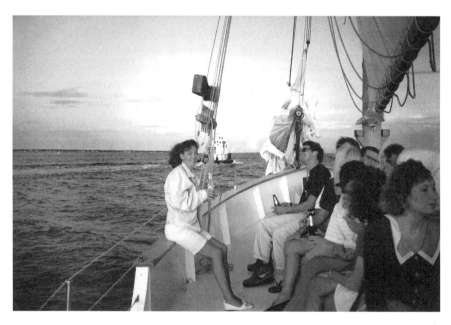

Sailing in Charleston Harbor. *Courtesy of Student Programs, MUSC.*

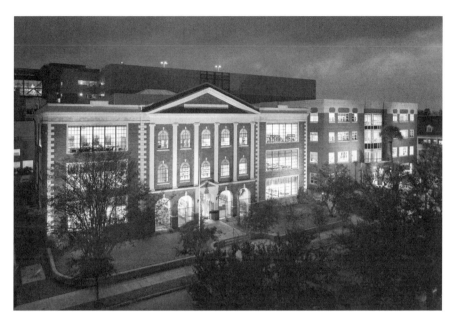

College of Health Professions Buildings at night. *Courtesy of College of Health Professions, MUSC.*

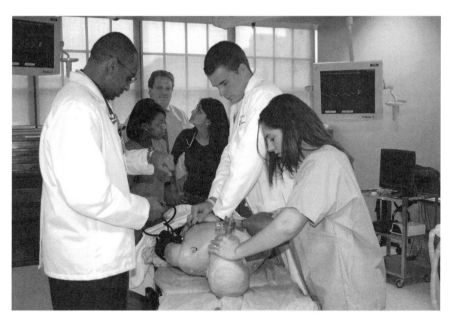

Physician assistant students in simulation lab. *Courtesy of College of Health Professions, MUSC.*

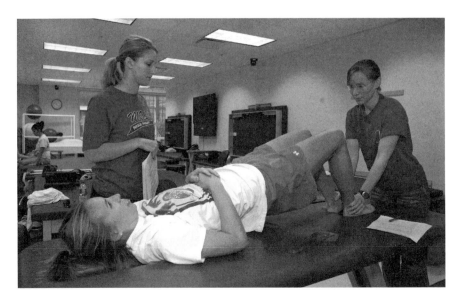

Physical therapy students in lab. *Courtesy of College of Health Professions, MUSC.*

one department is focused on education and the other on research; our goal is to have overlap between the two—research informing teaching and clinical situations leading research.

Our new initiative, the South Carolina Center for Rehabilitation Sciences, will focus on research in spinal cord injury, traumatic brain injury, traumatic amputation, and stroke. These are of special importance to South Carolinians because we are the "buckle of the stroke belt," and we also have an aging population and a high incidence of diabetes.

Emily E. Hardeman, in the master's degree program in Health Administration, 2009, explained her studies:

When you think about a health care administrator, you probably imagine somebody sitting at a computer pushing papers, handling billing or annoying caregivers about unnecessary costs. My experience has been very different. I joined the program to decide between the clinical and administrative side of medicine, to find out what career I wanted to pursue. On my third day of a ten-week internship at Bishop Gadsden, a continuing care retirement community, I think I may have already decided.

In the short time I have been here, I haven't spent much time behind a computer or knee-deep in paperwork. Instead, I have discovered hands-on administrative tasks by working with directors and clinicians who interact with residents in the community. Whether it is spending time in a resident's room or observing a directors' meeting, my time at Bishop Gadsden has shown me how interesting, rewarding and dynamic a career in long-term care can be.

The globalization that has occurred throughout MUSC is equally important for health professionals. Dr. Mark Sothmann, dean of the College of Health Professions, wrote from Hanzhou Province, China, in May 2009:

I am a long way from South Carolina this morning as I am here representing the College of Health Professions as part of the MUSC delegation to Jhejiang University in Hangzhou Province. Jhejiang University, the largest in China and one of its most prestigious in medicine, is building hospitals that will have a total capacity of over 6,500 beds—MUSC's hospital capacity is 650 beds. The university would like to partner with us in health administration; we would assist in building the operations of the new hospitals and educating their managers and leaders. This potential partnership follows similar discussions we have had with universities in India about educating hospital administrators for their booming healthcare infrastructure and for the future needs of their growing population. Opportunities on the international stage represent a next phase in CHP history.

GROSS ANATOMY STAYS LOCAL

Dr. Jack Thomas, professor in the division of physical therapy, is an award-winning teacher of gross anatomy, required for students in the physical therapy, occupational therapy and physician assistant programs. His description of his method revealed how the gross anatomy lab has changed over the years:

I have a large number of students in any gross anatomy lab. We work with prosections so at one station we might have a shoulder and a teaching assistant supervising a group of students, and at another an elbow. I try to create and maintain a friendly learning environment in which students rotate through all the stations, and I float, listening to their questions and interactions. Our approach to the body is regional, upper limb and back, and then lower limb, head and neck, chest and abdomen—the full body from head to toe. We do it all and it comes out pretty well.

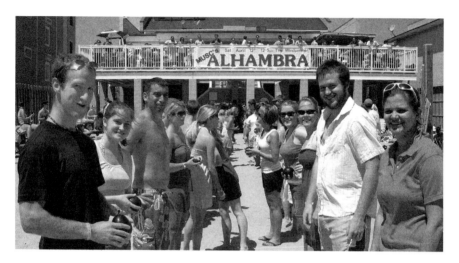

Annual Alhambra party. *Courtesy of Student Programs, MUSC.*

He remembered one student who made special demands:

> One of our female PT [physician assistant] students saw me walking across
> campus with my lab coat slung over my shoulder and wearing sunglasses. She
> said, "There goes Dr. Thomas. He's a real stud dog."...Later she got engaged
> and her friends gave her a bachelorette party at a restaurant and they set up
> a fake medical emergency. That's when I came in, bare chested in a lab coat
> and stethoscope with a Big Dog necktie...They handcuffed her to me. The
> place went wild. It was all over campus the next day, and I decided I had to
> rethink deals like that. But we're a very close bunch in this college.

CADAVERS GET RESPECT

The Humanities Committee was established in 1978 "to devise means for
integrating the humanities more fully with the total educational program at
MUSC." In 1996, the committee began publishing an annual literary magazine,
Humanitas. One of the essays in the first issue was written for the memorial
service held annually in St. Luke's Chapel to honor those who have donated their
bodies for dissection. Dr. Nicholas Batley (class of 1998) mused:

> The first dead body I saw was my grandfather's...[It] looked horrific. He
> had died of cancer and his skin was stretched over the bones of his wasted

face and he wore a grin full of pain and suffering...The next time I saw a dead body was during an interview for medical school. As we entered the dissecting room I thought of my grandfather and wondered if I would feel the same repugnance I had felt twenty years earlier. I did...for about five seconds and then I was overcome with fascination for what I saw. Part of the arm of the body had been dissected and there, laid before me, was the incredible complexity of the human hand. Actually, I had no idea then just how complicated it is. Many many many many hours of painful studies have corrected that little misconception.

And so to gross anatomy at MUSC. I'll always remember the first day at the gross lab. We waited outside the room joking nervously, trying to be cool...I remember one of my lab partners who for just about the entire first lab stayed as far away from our cadaver as possible...What a contrast when just a couple of months later that same lab partner leans casually on her cadaver, nonchalantly picks up a coil of intestine and says jejunum, right? Seems like a transition from the terrifying to the mundane. But it has never been that, not mundane. I think that always at some level there was the awareness that these cadavers were once people...

We all know that these people were once living breathing, crying, laughing, angry, passionate people. That they gave a wonderful gift to

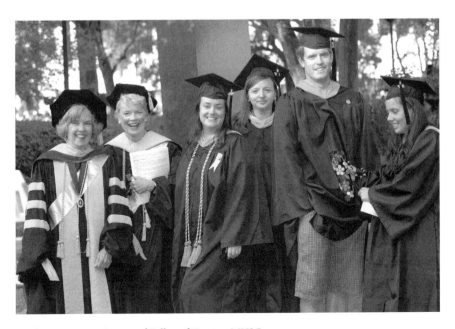

Graduation, 2007. *Courtesy of College of Nursing, MUSC.*

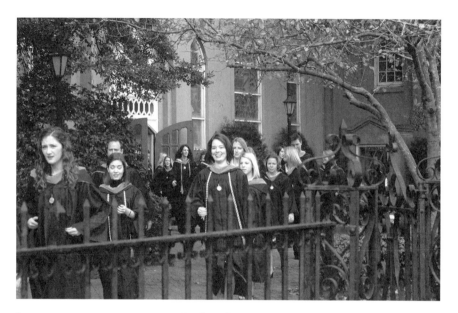

Leaving convocation, 2008. *Courtesy of College of Nursing, MUSC.*

a group of people whose predecessors had to rob graves for the same privilege we have enjoyed. AH! There's the rub, there's the point. It has been my rare privilege to dissect a human body and to the donors I offer two things: Firstly, a promise—to always honor their memory by trying to be the best doctor I can and secondly I offer my deepest thanks. Simply that, "Thank you."

MULTIPLE DEGREES FOR MEDICAL RESEARCHERS

The College of Graduate Studies was established in 1965 for students to earn masters' and PhD degrees in scientific fields and become biomedical research scientists. One of the courses of study is the combined MD/PhD, or the Medical Scientist Training Program. Andre Eaddy, a fifth-year student in 2009, explained why he entered this long—seven or eight years—and rigorous program:

My path to being a doctor was paved in stone until an unlikely hero, my eleventh-grade teacher, Mrs. Ginger Foley, opened my eyes to a different world, the world of scientific research. She encouraged me to apply to the

Experimental Program to Stimulate Competitive Research, sponsored by the Department of Energy. I developed an instant love of research.

A degree in biology from Morehouse College came next although when my mom asked, I still gave her the same answer. "Mom, I'm going to be a doctor." Somewhere along the way I even figured out that I could pursue both degrees, the medical degree and PhD in one sitting called an MD/PhD Program. I was going to cure cancer and heart disease and, as a pastime, save the planet. In a few years, a Nobel Prize would be within reach. Of course, no one told me where the "re" in re-search comes from. It comes from re-peat. I thought that when you discovered something, you discovered it. You know, Eureka! Right? Wrong! You actually have to discover something multiple times before anyone believes you. You need triplicates and duplicates and supplemental data, and controls (those endless experiments where you already know the answer and outcome but you have to do them and for some odd reason everyone wants to see those first). I didn't know that developing an "animal model" to simulate and study human disease really meant that I would be using some of the cutest little furry creatures ever. I didn't know that you essentially made your own schedule, meaning that you could take as many as ten years or as few as three years to finish your PhD.

I have completed the first two years of medical school, the first medical licensing exam and three years of graduate study of renal failure and cell death pathways—pathways important in most disease processes. Next I will finish the third and fourth years of medical school, then go on to a residency. The Nobel will come later.

CYBERSPACE AND EVIDENCE-BASED MEDICINE

As healthcare costs increased, healthcare providers needed to prove that the treatments they prescribed were actually effective. That meant looking at the evidence and keeping track of the evidence—a job for a librarian. Laura Cousineau, a librarian whose title is assistant director for program development and resource integration, explained the new practice known as evidence-based medicine and why librarians now make rounds:

> To be a good librarian, one needs a bloodhound's instinct to hunt down the answer to any question and a desire to satisfy every patron's information

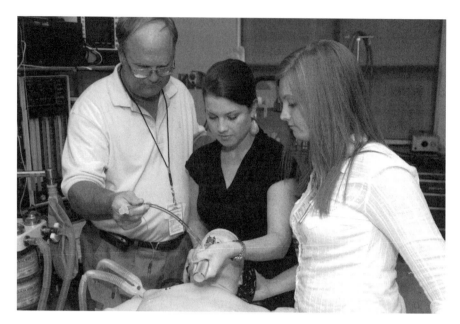

Anesthesia for nursing students in the simulation lab. *Courtesy of College of Health Professions, MUSC.*

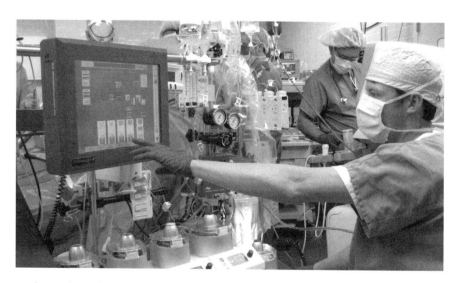

Cardiovascular perfusion student reading heart and lung monitors during open-heart surgery. *Courtesy of College of Health Professions, MUSC.*

need. Technology is the way we do that now. In the past we might have been acquiring papyrus scrolls or creating subject access headings for card catalogues, we are now buying e-journals and databases, and creating WIKIs, websites and podcasts. And in medical libraries, we are finding that place where our strengths in finding the right information intersect with healthcare providers' needs to treat patients based on the best medical evidence available. This is evidence-based medicine, or EBM.

EBM is a patient-oriented process that involves assessing the patient, forming a clinical question, searching for the best research article to answer the question, analyzing the article for validity and choosing proven approaches with the consent of and respect for the patient's situation and values. As a librarian, I teach EBM to students and healthcare providers, including how to analyze research articles and calculate the statistical values. I also participate on rounds, to help prompt questions, and develop a search strategy for finding the best evidence.

For medical librarians, this is juicy stuff. It is one thing to teach how to search a database, but quite another to be at the patient's bedside and positively contribute to that patient's optimal care. It makes us a real part of the healthcare team. And it motivates our quest—both the librarian's and the healthcare provider's—for lifelong learning.

SIMULATED BODIES FOR TWENTY-FIRST-CENTURY STUDENTS

The dentists have used plastic teeth for a long time, but the College of Nursing led the way in teaching students with complete simulated patients. Nicholas James Porter entered the College of Nursing in the fall of 2008 and immediately started posting a blog called "Naughty Mursing." (A murse is a male nurse.)

16 August 2008
...On Monday the 18th, my Orientation for the Accelerated BS in Nursing begins at MUSC, with classes starting on the 22nd. The most common question I've fielded thus far is, predictably, "Why?" Why in the hell would I, a college graduate and boxer with an alpha male complex, decide to enter nursing, a still overwhelmingly feminine profession and 180-degree turn from my English degree?

The short answer: Nursing Shortage.

The slightly less short answer: I need a goddamn job!

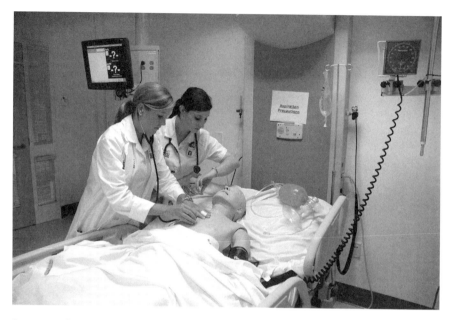

Sim man with nursing students in Sim Lab. *Courtesy of College of Nursing, MUSC.*

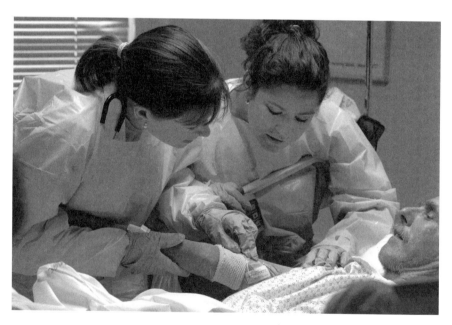

Nursing students with patient. *Courtesy of College of Nursing, MUSC.*

September 5 2008

Lesson from a mannequin in the Simulation Lab: if you are taking a patient's radial pulse and it stops, push into the wrist and the pulse will start again.

Lesson from a clinical instructor in the Simulation Lab: if a patient unexpectedly starts making screaming noises from the inside of his chest while blood pressure is being taken, put your hand over his mouth and reset his vital signs to the desired level.

Covering a patient's mouth when they scream unexpectedly is acceptable only if your patient is made of rubber.

AND YET, SOME VERY REAL PATIENTS

21 October 2008

In my short time, I've changed a dressing on a central line, which is a tube that leads directly to the vena cava and into the heart. I've learned to adjust ventilators that help people to breathe. I've learned how to assess patients, learning to look for things and knowing that my ability to do so could save a life. I held a patient's hand as she walked for the first time since a surgical procedure. In the ICU, as a patient came off of anesthesia and then slowly off of his ventilator, I literally had to remind him to breathe or, due to the anesthesia, he would forget.

And finally, a moment that will stick with me forever: A few weeks ago, I walked in to check on an elderly patient and found her in extreme pain, her husband at her side. She had headphones on, her TV was on: the distractions did nothing as she writhed in pain, tears in her eyes. I asked about her pain and her pain medication, then her husband took her headphones off, putting them around her neck. "Your hand doesn't hurt, does it? No? Okay then, focus on your hand," he said, as he slid his hand into hers. "Now focus on our hands together. We're going to be okay."

PLAYING DOCTOR

Dr. Melissa Matthews Fussell (class of 2009) recalled the doctoring curriculum and her training in "standardized patient care":

I peered down the corridor lined with exam room doors and found an awkward comfort in the wide-eyed looks of tension and anticipation on my classmates' faces. We stood shoulder to shoulder in a testing facility, built to resemble a doctor's office but functioning as a center where students meet actors impersonating patients. In the short white coats of fourth year medical students, we waited to take our standardized patient test, hoping the stethoscopes draped around our necks empowered us with the wisdom and pride of doctors.

Here I was, determined to treat my first "standardized patient." The sign on the door read, "eighty-one year old female with nausea and headaches," but the woman in the room was trained to portray a patient. She had been primed to emulate the appropriate symptoms, emotions, and physical findings. I wondered if it was possible to recreate the "perfect doctor-patient interaction" and feasible to learn diagnosing skills from a fabricated illness. No doubt, I had to remember the textbook chapters on nausea and headaches, but this exam and elaborate testing facility existed to evaluate my ability to comfort and heal a distressed and emotional human being.

I took a deep breath, knocked on the exam room door, entered, and saw my patient. She was a plump, grey haired woman, whose hospital gown meagerly protected her nudity from my naivety. She rustled the paper on the exam table, ready to perform the lines she had memorized. I stammered an introduction and asked what brought her in. She recited her case as I tried to remember the list of questions I was supposed to ask. Caught in the moment, I forgot to listen to her answer. I panicked. Had she just described her battle with indigestion or had she said she wanted to ask a question? I kept going and asked if she could tell me more about her reasons for coming.

Suddenly, a shadow stirred behind the darkened glass of the far wall, and I became painfully aware of the physician behind the two-way mirror, silently critiquing my doctoring techniques. I knew that he was checking my basic science knowledge, my lines of questioning, and my examination skills. And there was more. He was judging my compassion as a doctor and my empathy as a human being. I knew all the requirements, but I had only a few months of exposure to this vast world of medical knowledge.

I rushed through my memorized interrogation. My patient's confusion and hesitancy suggested that I had used the wrong line of questioning. Maybe I could redeem myself with the physical exam. Starting with her head, I dutifully remembered to look in her eyes, palpate her lymph nodes, and examine her ears, but then I battled clumsily with the otoscope. The

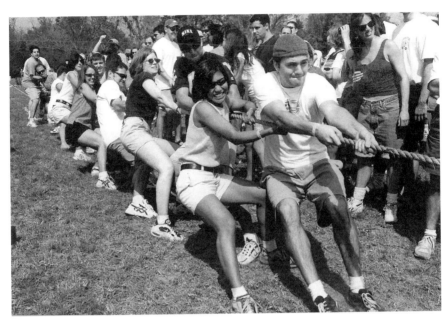

Traditional tug of war at Alhambra. *Courtesy of Student Programs, MUSC.*

plastic earpieces spilled across the exam room floor, the attachment failed to screw on properly, and then the plastic cone lodged in her ear. Trying not to laugh, my patient slowly removed it and handed it to me. As the catastrophe unfolded, I fumbled through the remainder of the exam, thanked the kind woman for her patience, and left the room with a defeated sigh.

My new doctor pride was momentarily lost, but looking back, I realized that I had survived my first patient encounter, braved this expensive facility, and begun my transition from the frightened and unsure medical student to the skilled practitioner.

IN CONCLUSION

Dr. W. Curtis Worthington (class of 1953), professor emeritus of anatomy, is an avid historian and director of the Waring Historical Library. In an interview for the College of Medicine Annual Report, he offered this summary:

> The College of Medicine is among the oldest medical schools in the United States. My contention is that it is the sixth oldest continuously existing

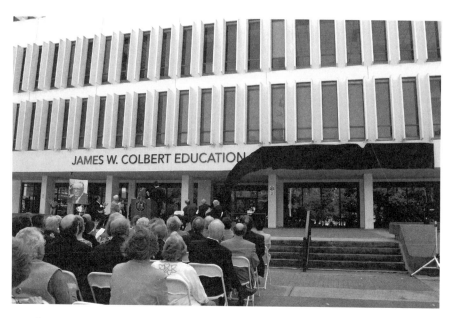

Unveiling the new name: James W. Colbert Education Center and Library, 2009. *Courtesy of Office of Public Relations, MUSC.*

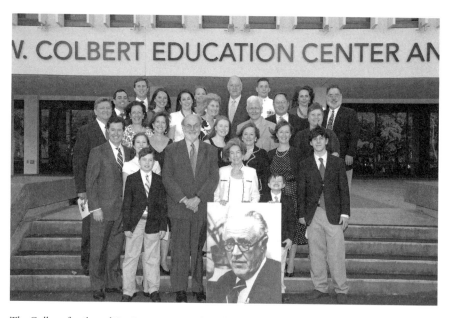

The Colbert family and Dr. Layton McCurdy in front of the James W Colbert Education Center and Library, 2009. *Courtesy of Office of Public Relations, MUSC.*

medical faculty in the United States and the oldest south of Baltimore. Its tenacity is unique. Throughout the College's history, people have fought for it! They fought to get it started and won. They fought for survival after the Civil War and within six months of Lee's surrender at Appomattox, the College was once again educating physicians. They faced extinction again after the earthquake in 1886 and rebuilt. Former dean, Robert Wilson, M.D. fought to upgrade medical education by becoming a state-funded university, and after a hotly contested debate, secured a victory for the College on a 25 to 14 vote by the [State of South Carolina] Senate...Regardless of what history threw its way, the College has maintained its integrity and held fast to its job of training physicians for South Carolina.

In April 2009, the library building at MUSC was renamed the James W. Colbert Education Center and Library. Dr. Colbert's famous son, Stephen Colbert—actor, writer, TV personality—remembered his father:

> My father was tall with a scratchy face and smelled like cigarettes. He loved fishing and he loved reading—especially French philosophers like Jacques Maritain. His favorite movie was *Hospital*—when someone says, "This place has gone to hell," and the George C. Scott character says, "Someone is responsible." That was his "the buck stops here."
>
> He would be very happy about his name on this building if only because it makes my mother happy, but also because he really loved education—especially research and learning. The fact that it is an education center and library is especially fitting.

And as Stephen Colbert reminded all the graduates and their families in his 2009 commencement address, we need healthcare professionals—because we certainly don't want amateurs.

BIBLIOGRAPHY

MANUSCRIPT COLLECTIONS

Avery Research Center, College of Charleston.
———. Charleston Hospital Strike file.

Charleston County Public Library.
———. Medical University of South Carolina File.

Charleston Library Society.
———. Pamphlet Collection, 1845–46.

The Citadel Archives and Museum.
———. F.L. Parker Journal, 1861.

College of Charleston, Addlestone Library, Special Collections.
———. Dickson, Samuel Henry, MD. "Annual Report to the President and Board of Trustees of The Medical College of the State of South Carolina, with the Valedictory Address to the Class," Charleston, 1841.
———. Simons, Thomas Y., MD. "An Introductory Lecture, Delivered in The Medical College of South Carolina in November 1835."

South Carolina Historical Society.
———. Henry B. Horlbeck Papers, 1839–1901.
———. John L. Manning Papers, 1839–88.
———. Francis Peyre Porcher Papers, 1801–88.
———. Walter Peyre Porcher Papers, 1871–1919.
———. Dr. Edmund Ravenel Papers, 1820–71.
———. Joseph Talliaferro Taylor Papers, 1870–1943.

South Caroliniana Library, University of South Carolina.
———. William Andrew Carrigan Papers, 1844–89.
———. Rosslee Green Douglas Papers, 1938–2003.
———. Gaston, Strait, Wylie and Baskin Family Papers.
———. Francis Bernard Higgins Papers.
———. Jones, Watts and Davis Family Papers.

———. Edward Henry Kellers Papers, 1852–93.

———. Lebby Family Papers, 1826–1940.

———. Samuel Wells Leland Diaries.

———. Gabriel Manigault Autobiography (typescript).

———. Thomas Jefferson McKie Papers, 1844–78.

———. Ravenel Family Papers, 1757–1894.

———. Hilla Sheriff Papers, 1908–89.

———. Whetsone Family Papers.

Southern Historical Collection, University of North Carolina Library.

———. Battle Family Papers.

Waring Historical Library, Medical University of South Carolina.

———. Titre J. Beakerdram Poems, n.d.

———. Brown, Alton G., Sr., MD. "Memoirs of a Retired Surgeon and War Diaries," unpublished typescript, n.d.

———. Brown, Laurie L., MD. "Oral histories of physicians' reminiscences, mainly concerning their experiences in World War II and the Korean and Vietnamese conflicts," unpublished typescript (including reminiscences of Sol Neidich, Thomas Marion Davis, Harold E. Jervey and Frederick MacNaughton Ball).

———. Buhler, John E., DDS. Papers, 1923–72.

———. College of Nursing Collection, 1887—2006.

———. College of Nursing Ledgers (handwritten), 1915–22.

———. Cooper, Thomas, MD. "An Address Delivered Before the Medical Board of South Carolina at Columbia, December, 1821."

———. Elizabeth Cork, Diary, 1906.

———. Henry W. DeSaussure, Lecture Notes, 1867.

———. James B. Edwards Papers, 1982–99.

———. Robert Haskell Harper, Ledgers, 1914–15.

———. Theodore Hayne Papers, 1898–1930.

———. Henry Tracy Ivy, Diary, 1880.

———. William Mellon McCord, MD, PhD, Papers, 1964–75.

———. Medical College of the State of South Carolina. Thesis. Agnew, Enid. "On The morbid effects of Intemperance upon the Animal Economy," 1845.

———. Medical College of the State of South Carolina. Thesis. Eveleigh, Thomas. "On the Properties of the Xanthum Strumarium or Common Sheep Bur as an Antidote to The poison of Venemous Serpents," 1831.

———. Medical College of the State of South Carolina. Thesis. Hearst, John W. "The Properties, Uses and Injurious effects of Nicotiana Tabacum," 1836.

———. Medical College of the State of South Carolina. Thesis. Jones, Larkin G. "On The peculiarities of the Female, the physiological changes produced by Conception, and The treatment of some of the most important diseases consecutive to parturition," 1829.

———. Medical College of the State of South Carolina. Thesis. King, Courtney S. "Yellow Fever as it appeared in Charleston during the summer of 1852," 1853.

———. Medical College of the State of South Carolina. Thesis. McRee, Wm. Lucius. "On the use of Cold Water As a Therapeutic Agent," 1840.

———. Medical College of the State of South Carolina. Thesis. Pope, F. Perry. "On the Professional Management of Negro Slaves," 1837.

———. Minutes of the Faculty of the Medical School of South Carolina, 1824–25, 1872, 1894.

———. Minutes of the South Carolina Medical Society, November 22, 1822.

———. Columbus Morrison, Lecture Notes, Winter, 1827–28 from "Samuel Henry Dickson, Theory and Practice of Medicine."

———. William Cyril O'Driscoll, MD, Papers, 1865–1951.

———. James J. Palmer Diary.

———. Pamphlet Collection. Annual Announcement, Medical College of the State of South Carolina, 1882.

———. Pamphlet Collection. Annual Announcement, Medical College of the State of South Carolina, 1894.

———. Pamphlet Collection. Catalogue, Medical College of the State of South Carolina, 1899–1900.

———. Pamphlet Collection. James Moultrie Jr. MD. "Memorial on the State of Medical Education in South Carolina." 1835.

———. South Carolina Training School for Nurses, Charleston, S.C. 1883.

———. Elsie E. Taber, PhD, Papers, 1911–2000.

———. Robert Wilson, Dean's Records, 1899–1938.

Interviews by the Editors

Colbert, Stephen. May 2009.

Collins, Dr. Edward (Eddie). May 2009.

Deas, Dr. Bernard. April 2009.

Douglas, Rosslee Green. June 2008.

Edwards, Dr. James Burrows. May 2009.

Gazes, Dr. Peter C. May 2009.

Gibbs, Dr. Rose Delores. April 2009.

Golod, Dr. William H. March 2009.

Hodges, James. March 2009.

McCullough, Catherine. April 2009.

McCurdy, Dr. Layton. April 2009.

Othersen, Dr. H. Biemann, Jr. April 2009.

Pilcher, Dr. Elizabeth. May 2009.

Thomas, Dr. K. Jackson. May 2009.

Welsh, Dr. Edward (Ted) L. May 2009.

Wilkie, Dr. Ralph. January 2009.

PERIODICALS

Aesculapian. November 1909, October 1910.

Bulletin of the Medical Women's National Association. 1931.

The Catalyst (MUSC). 1982–2009.

Charleston Courier. April 12, 1866.

Charleston Evening Post. 1969, 1978.

The Charleston Medical Journal and Review. 1848.

Charleston Post and Courier. 1969, 2003.

Charleston Sunday News. 1913.

The Chart (MUSC). 1980–81.

Civil War Times Illustrated. 1965.

Confederate Veteran. 1914.

Horizon (College of Nursing). 1989.

Journal of the South Carolina Medical Association. August 1996, November 1987, March 1988.

Lifelines (College of Nursing). 2008.

The Mouthpiece (College of Dental Medicine). 1972.

New York Times. 1912, 1969.

The Prognosis (nursing student newsletter). 1973.

The Scribe of the Charleston Medical Society. 1956, 1958.

South Carolina Historical and Genealogical Magazine. 1911.

The State, Columbia. 1969.

BOOKS

Banov, Charles H. *Office Upstairs: A Doctor's Journey.* Charleston, SC: The History Press, 2007.

Baruch, Bernard M. *Baruch: My Own Story.* New York: Henry Holt and Co., 1957.

Baruch, Simon. *Lessons of a Half Century of Medicine.* Richmond, VA: Dominion Publishing Corp., 1910.

Bonner, Thomas Neville. *Becoming a Physician: Medical Education in Britain, France, Germany and the United States.* London: Oxford University Press, 1995.

Bonner, Walter. *A Doctor's Toughest Case: A Girl, a Disease, a Medical University.* Charleston, SC: The History Press, 2005.

Bryan, Charles S. *A Most Satisfactory Man: The Story of Theodore Brevard Hayne, Last Martyr of Yellow Fever.* Spartanburg, SC: Reprint Co., 1996.

Centennial Memorial of the Medical College of the State of South Carolina, 1824–1924. Charleston, SC: Medical College of the State of South Carolina, 1924.

Chaddock, Katherine E., and Carolyn B. Matalene. *College of Charleston Voices: Campus and Community Through the Centuries.* Charleston, SC: The History Press, 2006.

Chamberlin, Ruth. *The School of Nursing of the Medical College of South Carolina—Its Story.* Charleston, SC: MUSC Alumni Association, 1970.

Chisholm, J. Julian. *A Manual of Military Surgery for the Use of Surgeons in the Confederate Army.* Charleston, SC: Evans and Cogswell, 1861.

Flexner, Abraham. *Medical Education in the United States and Canada: A Report to the Carnegie Foundation for the Advancement of Teaching (Bulletin 4, 1910)*. New York: Arno Press, 1972 [circa 1910].

Jervey, Louis, and W. Curtis Worthington Jr. *The Medical Society of South Carolina: The First Two Hundred Years*. Charleston, SC: Medical Society of South Carolina, 1989.

Keil, Julian E., and Edwin Boyle. *His Clock Had No Hands: The Story of Edwin Boyle, Jr., M.D. and the Charleston Heart Study*. Charleston, SC: Medical University Press, n.d.

Kett, Joseph. *The Formation of the American Medical Profession: The Role of Institutions, 1780–1860*. New Haven, CT: Yale University Press, 1968.

Kilbride, Daniel. *An American Aristocracy: Southern Planters in Antebellum Philadelphia*. Columbia: University of South Carolina Press, 2006.

Kiley, John Cantwell. *The Heart of a Surgeon: The Life and Writings of Horace Gilbert Smithy, M.D., Heart Surgeon, 1914–1948*. Berryville, VA: J.C. Kiley, 1984.

Lynch, Kenneth M. *Medical Schooling in South Carolina, 1823–1969*, Columbia, SC: R.L. Bryan Co., 1970.

McCandless, Peter. *Moonlight, Magnolias, and Madness: Insanity in South Carolina from the Colonial Period to the Progressive Era*. Chapel Hill: University of North Carolina Press, 1996.

O'Brien, Ed Michael, and David Moltke-Hansen. *Intellectual Life in Antebellum Charleston*. Knoxville: University of Tennessee Press, 1986.

Ogier, Thomas Lewis. *Memoir of Dr. John Edwards Holbrook*. Charleston, SC: Walker, Evans and Cogswell, 1871.

Porcher, Francis Peyre. *Resources of the Southern Fields and Forests, Medical, Economical, and Agricultural*. Richmond, VA: Charles Evans and Cogswell, 1863.

Pratt-Thomas, H. Rawling. *From Yorkshire Pudding to Hominy Grits: Exhumation of a Pathologists Life*. Greenville, SC: Southern Historical Press, 2002.

Sims, J. Marion. *The Story of My Life*. New York: D. Appleton, 1885.

Stoddard, Belle Howe. *Gedney Main Howe, Jr.* Adamsville, AL: Action Printing Co., 1985.

Stowe, Steven. *Doctoring the South: Southern Physicians and Everyday Medicine in the Nineteenth Century*. Chapel Hill: University of North Carolina Press, 2004.

Sunderman, James, and Jacob Rhette Motte. *Journey Into the Wilderness: An Army Surgeon's Account of Life in Camp*. Gainesville: University of Florida Press, 1963.

Ward, Patricia S. *Simon Baruch: Rebel in the Ranks of Medicine, 1840–1921*. Tuscaloosa: University of Alabama Press, 1994.

Waring, Joseph Ioor. *A History of Medicine in South Carolina, 1670–1825*. Charleston: South Carolina Medical Association, 1964.

———. *A History of Medicine in South Carolina, 1825–1900*. Charleston: South Carolina Medical Association, 1967.

———. *A History of Medicine in South Carolina, 1900–1970*. Charleston: South Carolina Medical Association, 1971.

Worthington, W. Curtis, H. Rawling Pratt-Thomas and Warren A. Sawyer. *A Family Album: Men Who Made the Medical Center*. Spartanburg, SC: Reprint Co., 1991.

Wragg, William T. *Memoir of Dr. James Moultrie*. Charleston, SC: William G. Mazyck, 1869.

ABOUT THE EDITORS

This is the third collaborative book tracing the history of institutions of higher education by these authors. Their earlier works were *Carolina Voices: Two Hundred Years of Student Experiences* and *College of Charleston Voices: Campus and Community Through the Centuries*. Both authors live in Charleston.

Carolyn B. Matalene taught for many years in the English department at the University of South Carolina, specializing in composition and rhetoric. Her research appears in *Worlds of Writing, Professional Writing in Context, Telling Stories/Taking Risks* and numerous journals. She was the 1998 recipient of the University of South Carolina's Amoco Outstanding Teaching Award and is now a distinguished professor emerita.

Katherine E. Chaddock is a professor and department chair in the College of Education, University of South Carolina. Her teaching and research emphasizes the history and administration of higher education. She is the author of dozens of scholarly articles and chapters as well as five books, including *Visions and Vanities: John Andrew Rice of Black Mountain College* and (with Susan Schramm) *A Separate Sisterhood: Women Who Shaped Education in the Progressive Era*.